To CAMEASHA

thanks for your support

Darrell Barkley

Remember

Don't Suffer In Silence

www.myspace.com/thebarkleygroup

Heart Broken Soulmate

Randell W. Barkley

Bloomington, IN Milton Keynes, UK

AuthorHouse™
1663 Liberty Drive, Suite 200
Bloomington, IN 47403
www.authorhouse.com
Phone: 1-800-839-8640

AuthorHouse™ UK Ltd.
500 Avebury Boulevard
Central Milton Keynes, MK9 2BE
www.authorhouse.co.uk
Phone: 08001974150

This book is a work of non-fiction. Unless otherwise noted, the author and the publisher make no explicit guarantees as to the accuracy of the information contained in this book and in some cases, names of people and places have been altered to protect their privacy.

© 2007 Randell W. Barkley. All rights reserved.

No part of this book may be reproduced, stored in a retrieval system, or transmitted by any means without the written permission of the author.

First published by AuthorHouse 4/24/2007

ISBN: 978-1-4259-8724-4 (sc)

Library of Congress Control Number: 2006911203

Printed in the United States of America
Bloomington, Indiana

This book is printed on acid-free paper.

Dedications

I dedicate this book to my wife, Sonita Barkley and our children, Jehdiah, Josiah, Abijah, Shereef and the unborn.

May y'all rest in peace.

CONTENTS

Introduction		*xi*
One	*The Move*	1
Two	*Those Eyes*	9
Three	*The Conspiracy*	17
Four	*Reunited*	28
Five	*Jersey Bound*	40
Six	*First Born*	57
Seven	*The Departure.*	78
Eight	*Third Child*	119
Nine	*Spiritual Test*	134
Ten	*Marriage*	150
Eleven	*Fourth Child*	182
Twelve	*The Unthinkable*	200

Acknowledgments

I would like to thank my business consultant, Kareem Ali For believing in me, and helping me stay focus on the important of my book. Thank you for your loving support.

I would also like to thank my editor, Mrs. Chappell for seeing the vision, and bringing out the best in me.

I would also like to thank my children, Sean, Naquasha, Randell Jr. and Rhashon Barkley, who stuck by me through the time it took to complete my book. I appreciate y'all patience with me. I love y'all dearly.

I can't forget the many women who shared their life experiences with me at the times when I wanted to quit. Thank you for encouraging me to continue on bringing light about this issue women deal with in silence.

I would like to thank my first wife, Susan Perry for comforting me through the most fragile state I have ever endured. We are forever one.

I would like to thank Danielle Hutchinson for bringing me a new life in this world, Jahmae' Barkley. Three years after my tragedy. Thank you for helping me feel loved again.

I can't forget my brother's Dawu, Kasseem, Ibn, Khalif, Majid, Mahammed, Yah'Yah, Quadir, and my sister's, Sherone, Christie, Katrina, Fatima, and Kyla who held me down when I no longer wanted to be around. Thank you for being there for me.

I also like to thank the Jehovah's Witnesses who help me see and realize the love Jehovah has for all mankind, and I appreciate y'all loving spiritual support.

I can't forget the number 1 sound in VA, King Eternity, for supporting and strengthen me through hard times.

I also would like to thank William Otey, Eric Loney, Christopher Parks, Jed, and Spoon for ya'll support.

I would like to thank my cousins, Thomas, Rah-Baldie, Jamil, and Alimu for reaching out to me from prison, yah have giving me the strength and will to beat the odds and never give up. Thank you for your example of strong will and faith.

Last but definitely not least, I got to give an unconditional shot out to my cousin Keisha and her daughter Marshae for saving my life,

I wouldn't be alive if it wasn't for you. One Love.

To all others who I may have forgot, thank you all for showing me your loving support.

Introduction

September 29, 2002. My wife, Sonita Barkley murdered three of our children.

She jumped off of the Campostella Bridge; killing herself and her unborn child. The local media immediately figured that I, Randell Barkley, was the cause for this tragedy.

Insinuations flared that I either drove her to that point, or she was in an abusive relationship and felt this was her only way out. However, it's not true. I'm writing this book to shed light on the real her, Sonita Barkley, my soul mate.

Sonita was a very loving, caring, and spiritual, out going, exciting person. She was not crazy. So how could this be the end? What was she going through inside. You will be shock to know how a person childhood can effect their adulthood. Depression is a silent killer that society still doesn't view in its entirety. Hopefully this book will help people see how the common things we live with can have a diverse effect from one person to the next.

As you peer into the life of my two wives and me, I hope you grasp something that can help you discern the best decision to make in your life. You may have an aunt, a mom, a sister, a cousin, or friend dealing with *Post Partum Depression* or *Post Partum Psychosis*. If so, this book may help them see the signs and hopefully take advantage of the limited health organizations *now* available to help women.

On your journey in my world please have an open mind and a sincere heart as you digest Sonita, Susan, and I reality.

ONE
The Move

In April of 1993, I was 23 years old and I lived on Main st in East Orange New Jersey. It's a small town next to Newark New Jersey. I worked at African Techniques Barber shop. The shop was very afro centric. It consists of four barbers and one hair braider. It was a fun time in my life because I had recently gotten release from jail six months ago and my friend Jay got me a job at this shop. I married my first wife, Susan Perry on July 13, 1991, and we had three children during this union. Sean he's 7, my daughter Naquasha who was 4, and Randell Jr who was 2 years old. I loved her and my children very much, but we were going through a lot of changes. We were from two different places and it was hard to adjust. Another fact was, we got married too young and for the wrong reasons. I married her, basically because she had my babies. I really didn't know her at all. I thought that was the right thing to do. However time proved otherwise. Quite a number of girls pursued me, so I was unfaithful to my wife, and as a result my wife was also. Once we admitted to each other what we were doing we broke up. She ended up moving back to Brooklyn New York, and I stayed in East Orange, New Jersey.

My house became the fun house. I had the living room turn into a dance floor.

The dining room was the social area, and the 3 bedrooms were for the wild people.

We partied, got high, and performed sexual acts every weekend. From time to time I would be with my family in Brooklyn. There was no hope for Susan and me getting back together now.

Meanwhile my boss Jeffrey decided to move his business to Virginia Beach Virginia. So, that put the other barbers and me out of business. We didn't know what to do. Saturday we were just at work. Monday when we come to work, our boss packed up the whole shop, and was moving down South.

Two of the barbers went to High st. down in Newark to cut hair. The other barber went to a shop close to where he lived at over in South Orange New Jersey.

I had no shop to go to, so I had to think fast. I put a sign on the old shop telling people to come to my house for service. I just so happened to live four stores down on the third floor. My landlord, (Kim) had her Korean boutique on the first floor. It was a salon on the second floor owned by an African lady (Akeara). Now, I was on the top floor by myself. I turned my dining room into my barber shop and customers waited in my living room. My little brother, Teric, had the back room. We turned my other bedroom into a game room and it was on from there!

My place could hold 40 people easy. I called Jay and told him to cut hair with me because everyone was coming to my house and I couldn't handle the overflow of customers.

In the meantime the African lady on the second floor noticed all the traffic I was having and due to the fact her business wasn't doing too well, she offered me her shop.

I thought for a minute and figured that I could double that number easy in her place.

I ran the idea to a customer I had known about four months now.

He was a cool, Jamaican kid, I pick up packs from. He said," Love, that's a great idea. How much do she want for de shop?"

I told him" $16,000.00." He then responded,

"Word love; let me be your partner. When you finish with me cut, come to me truck."

I said bet. His truck was park out side across the street from the shop.

When we get to his truck he gave me $10,000.00 in cash out of a black leather bag.

He then said, "Love have her draw up de contract. You put de six to it and give me my two grand me fronting you when me get back seen." He turn and began to get in his truck.

I yelled,"Yo where are you going?" He replied,

"To Arizona for two months." I said to him, "So you gonna trust me with all this money?" He said,

"Yes, me know you gonna do de right ting. (Smile)"

It was all good. I hired Jay, YahYah, Rasheen, my cousin Keisha and three of her friends.

Everybody was straight. I flipped $5,000.00 and gave Akeara $5,000.00 at the end of the first month, I paid her $11,000.00 I was sitting on $5,000.00 I decided to throw myself a big New Years Eve Party.

1994 rolled around and my partner was back. It was all good between us.

I met this girl name Keisha in my shop, and we hit it off as she walk in from the door.

She was fine. Light skinned hazel eyes with a pretty petite shape.

We began to live the life. Then, I got her pregnant and all hell broke loose. My wife found out and she was pregnant also. They had an altercation and the stress of it caused Keisha to lose the baby she was carrying.

My younger cousins got into big trouble and they were looking at spending life in prison. I was trying to help them the best way that I could. My uncle came home from prison and while we were together, he became involved in a shoot out and killed somebody. After that, I get into a car accident and totaled my jeep. Later on my partner tells me he has to go out of town again and said he would be back within a month. Meanwhile, the other barbers in my shop were talking with the

Korean guy who owns the shop we left, and he offered them a job and they accepted.

I really didn't mind because they were running over me, plus they never paid their booth rent on time. They figured we were boys so why respect me as the boss.

Jealousy is deadly.

Some crazy shit happened to my partner while he was away.

He stopped calling me like he used to and then all of a sudden, the Jamaican Mob started coming by looking for him. It was one slim guy with a low cut and two big dudes with dreads. The slim guy started questioning me about things I knew nothing about. I snapped on him and said that whatever they had going on with him didn't concern me, so leave me the fuck alone! I went out and bought me a bullet proof vest and I kept my nine millimeter on my side.

Meanwhile, my brother Samad calls me from V.A. He says, "Yo Hakeem I got it going on and I want you to come and visit me in April." It was the beginning of March so I said" cool it was getting hectic up here anyway." I let my apartment go and I moved in with Keisha. That way I could get away from the shop at night.

Later on, the FBI came to the shop looking for my partner. I told them the same thing I told the mob, "I don't know anything."

A week before April came around and this guy named Weezy came to the shop with my brother Dawoo." He looked around the shop and said, A Hakeem, I like your shop, your father used to cut my hair, and as a result he inspired me to become a barber. You know, I got a shop down in V.A., so if you decided to come down there you could go into business with me."

I said," word, my brother Samad is down there, next week I'm going to visit him."

"That's peace Hakeem, what are you doing after work?"

"Nothing."

Dawoo said" Why don't you go with us to New York?

We are going to get high off of everything."

I said," bet."

We left and I had a good time. We were so fucked up; we got lost and couldn't find our way home until the next day.

Meanwhile, it was time for me to go to V.A. I caught the Grey Hound bus down there, and a cab to the spot in Norfolk V.A. where Samad was. My other brother Teric moved down there new years that just passed. I couldn't Waite to see him.

When I get to Samad spot there's an AK- 47 lying around, pump sawed-off shotguns, Tech Nines and 44 Magnums. I said," This is where you stay?" He said,

"One of the places." They had pounds of weed everywhere. I said," Fuck this Teric, take me to your mother's house! "They laugh and Samad said" it's not like home, it's alright."

"I said," No its not, this looks like a spot up in New York and I don't want to be here."

Samad looked at me and said,

"I respect that. Teric take Love to your mother's house when I get off at 12:00 midnight I'll come get him." He introduced me to his friends, like Big Teric, Vlady, Treyindo, and Swinger.

We waited until the cab came and we bounce…

I saw Teric's mom and we played cards, ate her famous home cook chicken, drunk beer, and smoked weed. Samad came by and we went to his apartment.

Big Teric, Swinger, Dread, and Due were there and they all was playing play station.

The house was so flooded with smoke, it took me a minute to realize I knew Due and Dread from the Bricks and I was happy to see them. Dread put on weight and he was growing his Locks, a college student doing his thing. Due took me out on the town.

We were just alike; the dressy type that love's to party and be around women. Samad knew that; That's why he hooked me up to go out with Due the first night I got down there and I had a ball! We got back to Samad's house around 4:00 am. They were still up smoking weed. I was shocked. I said to myself, either that's some garbage ass weed or you jokers are addicts.

The next day, when I wake up, they are handing me a blunt.

I said" Damn where is the hospitality at? I thought in the South y'all had the grits and eggs cooking? The first thing you hand me is a blunt? Where is the nearest store, I need some food."

I went to Kentucky Fried Chicken. I ordered a three piece, with mash potatoes and macaroni and cheese for my sides. After that we played basketball and I met Kirk.

He was cool as hell. That night was the Grand opening for their club called Diamonds; it was in Chesapeake V.A. I threw on the outfit I bought and I partied all night long in V.I.P. style. I met Cooley, DaddyRuff and 45 that night. I had so much fun.

Because it was my birthday time and I was living it up to the fullest.

The next night we went to another club called The Broadway. However, we end up back at Diamonds for the night. I really enjoyed myself and I was very happy to see Samad doing well. He had a rough life up top and to see him excel and have his own, made me very proud of him.

The weekend went so fast; it was now time for me to go. I thanked Samad and his clique' for showing me unconditional love.

I told Samad that I'll be back here for good in six months.

I returned home and dealt with all my issues.

While my partner was unable to be found, my money was getting tight. Keisha didn't want to be bothered with me anymore. I wasn't dealing with my wife anymore, but I still went to see the children and give her support money. She just gave birth to my son Rahshon Khalif Barkley on July 19, 1994. The kid, Weezey, was calling me to tell me that I could go into business with him. Therefore, I sold the shop and bounced to V.A. in September of 1994.

Kiesha ended up coming with me to check things out for herself. She wanted a new start also she said.

I believed she just wanted to see if I had somebody down here already, but I didn't.

She bounced after a week and I began living with Teric and his mother. I kept calling Weezey so I could link with him, but he wouldn't return my calls and I started getting frustrated. I've been down here two weeks already and I have no job. Samad told me,

"if you want, you could run one of my spots; I'll pay you good Hakeem.

You could stay high, party and have all the sex you want." I told him,

"That's cool fam, but I got to at least try to make it on my own, my way and should I fail, then I'll be glad to." Samad hugged me and said,

"Well that's peace." Later that night, Weezey called me and ask if I would come past the shop in the morning. I agreed. Samad and I arrived the next morning. The size of the shop was nice. It wasn't as big as mine though, but I saw the potential. Weezey was there with his brother B, and another barber named Larry.

We all clicked, and then Samad left.

Weezey told him that he would take me home. I set my clippers up at the station and I began to cut my hair. Ego tripping showing off my skills. As the customers watched, they told Weezey that they wanted me to cut their hair. After 2 hours has passed, an old man came in the shop and started screaming. "Who the fuck is this you got cutting up in my barbershop Weezey?!? Is you fucking crazy?!?" Weezey said calmly, "Dad this is Hakeem from Jersey, Dawoo brother."

The man replied with anger" I don't give a fuck who's brother he is, or where the fuck he's from, I want him out my motherfucking shop right now!"

I said," Weezey I thought this was your shop!?"

The man said," Weezey's shop? I ought to throw your ass out with him!" Then, the man reached for his gun. I said," it's been a terrible mistake, but I'll leave. Calm the fuck down sir. You can put the gun away." I was scared out my wits, but I was playing it as cool as possible. I understood totally where he was coming from. Then, Weezey said," hold up Hakeem, I'm sorry for not telling you; it really is my father's shop. I wanted you to come down so you could give me some help, because my clientele is big, and they refuse to go to any one else. I knew that after they saw you cut, they would go to you, and that would help me." His father calmed down after Weezey had said his intention and then, he apoligized to me.

He explained that he wasn't mad at me, he was mad at his son for doing what he did without consulting him. All in all, everyone understood and we all went to the back of the shop to talk. I got the job, but I was mad as hell because Weezey had me under the assumption that we were going into business together, now I'm working for somebody.

I just sold my shop back in New Jersey.

I had 6 employees, and was making $2,000.00 a week.

Now, I'm dropping to $400.00 a week. That meant all my dough I brought down here with me is going to bills. I won't be able to invest and get my return, plus some!

I went out and found me a one-bedroom, instead of the three-bedroom condo I wanted.

I worked part time with Samad, to get some extra dough, and I was partying and doing me, player style to the fullest.

TWO
Those Eyes

MEANWHILE IN OCTOBER, IT was a beautiful afternoon day when three girls came into the barbershop. One of them was for Weezey, the other one was for Larry and the third girl was available. It was between B and me to get at her.

I didn't want to compete with him so I figured I let him shoot his game first; if she rolled with him, then I'll try to get with one of their other friends.

Anyway, I was really digging the girl who Weezey started talking to. She was the cutest of the three; Weezey set it up to get with them after work; however, he was on another mission, which included weed and coke and nothing else, so the following day they came by. Weezey was so ripped from last night he didn't even come in to work. Larry hollered for the girl he wanted and B did the same. The girl who was there for Weezey asked me, "What's your name?"

I said "Hakeem, and what's yours?" She replied,

"Janell." I said,

"That's pretty, my first name is Randell, it kind of rhymes. However, everyone calls me Hakeem." She and I end up kicking it. Then they left and said they would be back. Finally, Weezey made it in to work. Larry told him,"Yo Hakeem pulled your girl."

He said, "word" I said, and We suppose to link up tonight." He didn't even care; all he wanted was to make some money so that he could get high. When she came back, we went out to eat and had fun; then she dropped me off at home.

The following night, I left the shop early because Samad needed me in the spot.

While I was chilling with my peoples, someone said, "Hakeem, someone is here to see you." I thought they were joking, so I said,"yeah right." Then, I heard a girl's voice, so I went to the front and it was Janell. I said,

"How did you know where I was at?"

She said, "Weezey showed me, so I bounced with her and we went back to my house and chilled. The next week she came by and said, "Hakeem, I got to talk to you." I replied, "what's up?" Then she sobbed, "My sister got into some trouble and she needs a place to hide out, temporarily. Let me get the keys to your place and we will stay there until you get off from work. I'll come and pick you up later."

I said, Okay It was about 2 hours before she came back with her sister.

I was cutting hair at the time so I didn't notice Janell when she first came in; however, when her sister came in after her, and we caught eyes my heart jumped.

I said to myself, that's my new wife; I got to have her.

She tried to have a mean face, but I saw right through it and knew she was innocent and sweet.

The next thing that came to my mind was, how am I gonna get past her sister?

I finished cutting and I walked over to them. Janell introduced us, she spoke but she had an attitude.

I gave Janell my keys and said," They cut my lights off so pick up some candles." I joked about it for a minute. I couldn't believe how high my light bill was back in Jersey and it never got cut off.

My bill was change compared to it and they cut me off for $ 60.00 and Sonita laughed.

While they waited around I kept catching Sonita's eyes. Plus her beautiful smile. I fell in love with her at that moment, and I didn't know her at all. Janell told me, "we will be back later.

That night when they picked me up, on the ride Janell told me to talk to her because our lives were the same in many ways, and maybe I could give her some advice.

Once we got back to the house, we talked about her situation. Three girls jumped her and she pulled out a blade and sliced them up real bad. The police were looking for her and she didn't have no place to go. I felt real bad for her because she didn't have anyone to lean on, or be there for her. Janell was making it seem like the best thing for her to do would be to turn herself in. But, Sonita wanted to go to Hawaii with her sister Kim, or to Maryland with her cousin named Billy. She wasn't trying to go to jail. I didn't blame her, my mentality was "I'll pay up when they catch up." That night, Sonita crash on my couch while Janell and I were in my room.

We just talked the night away and eventually went to sleep.

The next morning I had to go to work, so I was rolling me up my morning blunt. Sonita wanted to smoke with me, but Janell said no then Sonita got mad and said," you only brought me here so you could be with him; shit, I haven't seen you in months."

I said" Shorty your sister said no and I can't override that." Sonita said,

"Well I'll be back on my own." Then Janell said" I don't think so, come on let's go."

We got in the car and bounced.

Janell stop to get some gas. While Janell pumped the gas I told Sonita," Look shorty if you need my help, come check me; I'll be here for you and that's my word is bond."

Janell got back in the car and took me to work. She told me she was going to be with her sister and she will check me later. I walked in the shop and everybody just stared at me. "What's up?"

Weezey said," I know you didn't hit both of them!"

I said, "No, I haven't hit neither one yet." (smile) In my mind I was hoping to see Sonita again.

I work the rest of the day and bounce to Samad's spot. I met this girl named Latonya there, we left, went to my house and fucked all night. The next day I went to work and Weezey told me that Janell came by. I said," word , what did she say?" She told him that she would be back.

Later on that day she came back. I walked outside to talk with her. She said, "I can't see you no more because my husband is coming back." I said,

"That's peace, I don't want no beef, being friends is fine with me." Then I asked her,

"What's up with your sister?" She looked puzzled and said "What do you mean what's up?" I replied "Is she alright?" optimistically she said,

"Yeah, she's fine. We are going to send her to Hawaii with our older sister." I said,

"Word I'm glad everything worked out for her." She then drove off.

I went back into the shop to tell the fellas about the girl named Latonya I fucked last night. I had them rolling.

I didn't see Janell any more after that. It really didn't matter to me because I had girls who was bout it bout it.

November rolled around and I had a ball the whole month.

It was Weezey, Larry, Samad, Lil Teric, Treyindo and I. My apartment stayed packed with women, beer, guns and drugs. We always partied at Diamonds on the weekends and ran the women to my apartment afterwards.

By the time December rolled around, I was partied out. I felt like I'd done everything I wanted to do. I had a little dough saved, I met mad good people, I was shining at work, but something was missing... My family; me hearing daddy, being a father and husband. I was straight, but I knew my wife wasn't. I knew it was harder to live in Brooklyn than it was in VA besides she was staying with her moms in a room with four of my children. I went to Newark New Jersey and told my mother what I wanted to do. She said" That would be the right thing to do for your children, but is that what Susan want? You know how she is plus y'all took each other through a world of pain. She looked at me and said,

"I'm a woman son and it may not be that easy for her to put them things behind. She's not going to trust you because she has been scarred. You may want to see if she would give you the children on the holidays and when they are out of school. That way you could build a rapport with your children, without any distractions. However, if you choose to bring her down there where you at, you know the first girl she see's you around, she's gonna feel that you are doing them, and there will be drama." I said,

"You're right mom, but I'm gonna give it a shot." I called Susan on the phone and she had an attitude. The children were stressing her out, plus her mother didn't make it any better. She was mad at her mother because she wanted her own space, plus she was dealing with a man.

I felt like Susan was jealous. Her mother had every right to be the way she was because Susan was grown and she really wasn't trying to do anything for herself. I suggested to Susan "lets start all over in VA You and our children can live with me .

I have my own apartment and it can just be us." She became quiet for a minute, then she said, "Are you serious?" I said "Yes." She said, "When is you talking about?" I said "Right now." She started crying on the telephone and said" okay." Then I told her,

"Look I was fucking while I was down there but I'm not messing with anyone now.

I want to start brand new with you. I don't care about who you been fucking with in Brooklyn or New Jersey.

Let's leave it there and go on." She said "Bet." I told her that I'll be there tomorrow to pick her and the children up. I hung up the phone and told my mother she said yes. My mother looked at me and said "Good luck son. I wish y'all the best, but it's not going to be easy."

The next day I moved my family from Brooklyn to VA with no car or help. I carried bags of clothes to the train, off the train to the greyhound bus, and from the greyhound bus, to a cab to my apartment in VA. My body was killing me, but I got my whole family down south. My wife, Sean, Naquasha, Randell jr, Rahshon and me.

They loved it down here. The first five days were beautiful.

The sixth day was a Thursday and there was a knock at the door, and my wife answered it. There was a girl I met a month ago named Sandy. She was cute, short, and petite with red hair. My wife figured that I hit it. However, I didn't. We kissed and caressed before, but the red lady was present so we didn't fuck. Afterwards when we got to know each other , we didn't want to. I told her about my plans to get my wife so she wanted to meet her to see whether she could help her get a job.

Susan said, "Who is this?" I said, "A friend I want you to meet and no I didn't have sex with her." I further explained,

"She lives down the block, so she can help you find a job while I'm at work." They met, then Sandy left. Susan sizes her up and gives her that look like, it better be true or I'm a fuck you up. I can tell Sandy caught that vibe too. That night Susan wouldn't let it rest. I had to tell her over and over I didn't have sex with Sandy. It's no way possible I'd have you meet a girl I had sex with.

So, Susan took it down.

The second week went by. Susan met Sandy's sister as we played cards and ate dinner.

I could tell Susan still wasn't feeling them because they were pretty girls and she knew they were my type. However, they were kind and cool as well. Her sister's children got along with ours, but Susan's guard was up. They also felt the vibe, but they overlooked it.

Meanwhile, my brother Teric and his mom lives across the hall in the other building. They came over and chilled with us. We had fun until Teric's adopted sister moved in because her boyfriend beat her up. Susan knew I did hit her when we were living in New Jersey and figured I would hit her again. I told Susan, "Look you've only been here for two weeks and you're buggin the fuck out. I don't want her no more, me and you are starting brand new. I know it's gonna take time to learn how to trust me, but damn give me the benefit of the doubt! If I wasn't trying to make it work, I would've left you in Brooklyn!" Then Susan softened up and said," You are right .

I am overreacting. I'm sorry."

Later that night I went out with Samad and got drunk as hell, therefore I couldn't make it home. When I get home the following day. Susan is mad as hell! She wouldn't let me in the house. Susan scream through the door "I know you was with Vanessa last night , that's why you didn't come home!" I shouted back at her,

"No, I wasn't I was with Samad! She screamed again,

"Go ahead and use Samad as your alibi, I don't believe you!!" I begged her to open the door; although she wouldn't, So I went over Teric's house and stayed over there for the next five hours.

When I knocked on the door this time she let me in.

The first thing she tells me to do is go into the bathroom. I go. Then she said, "Take your clothes off, I want to smell your dick." I yelled,

"What, are you crazy!" She exclaimed,

"If you didn't do nothing let me smell your dick now strip!"

She took me through her test." You passed this time, but I'm watching you."

At that moment there's a knock at the door. I go into the room to finally lay down. Then I hear Susan screaming my name,

Love, come here right now!! I get up and go to the door. Susan said," it's some girl at the door asking for you!!" I said, "what??? Who is she?" I open the door and it's Sonita. My heart jumps again as I stared into her pretty eyes. I said to myself ooh shit!

I spoke," hi, how are you doing long time no see. "

I then walked out the door to talk with her.

"What's up ? I haven't seen you in two months."

"I just escaped from this group home institution they had me in."

I said, "what? Your sister told me you went to Hawaii to live with your other sister."

"No, I didn't, Janell turn me in. I've been locked up since I saw you last.

I got this joker I don't even know, to bring me to your house.

My clothes and stuff is in his car." I whispered,

"Damn shorty, I got my wife and children living with me now." Her eyes started to water and she said,

"You gave me your word you would help me, plus it took us three hours to find you.

I couldn't really remember. I know this guy is gonna want some money from me, so what's up, can you help me or not?" I looked in her face and saw the sincerity of her words.

I said, "Fuck it. Yes, I gave you my word, get your stuff." She smiled and said,

"Hakeem, what about your wife?" I told her,

"Just listen, you are Weezey's cousin you're in some trouble and you don't want them to know. Weezey's father's name is Mr. Lensey his brother's name is B. Mr.lensey is your uncle, you got that?"

She said, "Yes." Now go get your stuff, I'm going to talk to my wife."

I thought damn, I'm already in the dog house it's really about to get worse. I went inside and told my wife the deal. I knew she couldn't refute it because she didn't know Weezey, his father or his brother. She just knew I worked for them. If she was their family the only thing I could do was help her.

I was letting her stay until I could talk to Mr. Lensey.

THREE
The Conspiracy

SONITA CAME IN AND I introduced her to my family. Susan was hot to death, but it was nothing she could do. She smelled and tasted my body then felt bad for accusing me. She had to trust me now.

By then it didn't matter to me, I just wanted to put a roof over shorty's head for now.

Susan was nice to her and also fed her. My children took to her automatically. I told her, I will help you get a place. But right now you got the living room. Good night." Sonita said "Hakeem thanks."

Then, we went to bed. I knew I had to put in work, so I made unconditional love to my wife and she fell to sleep. The next morning when we got up, the whole house was clean. The children were fed and she was braiding Rahshon's hair. I thought to myself. Shorty is a nice girl.

I was impressed, but Susan was heated. That Sunday I took her to meet Teric and Treyindo.

They came back to my house and Sonita braided Treyindo's hair.

It was the best braids he ever had. We all left to go to the store. Teric, Treyindo, Sonita, and me. I took the opportunity to talk with her one on one. I asked her,

"Where is your mother?" She put her head down and said,

"My moms died when I was 6 years old. My oldest sister name Kim raised me and my brother and two sister's." I felt sorry for her. I then asked her,

"Well, where is your father?"

She continued, "He was never there for me, I don't even know him. I mean, I know his name and my aunts told me he lived down the street from where we lived. However, he never came to see me." I was devastated. I had a lot of more questions I wanted to ask but I changed my mind.

Sonita began to talk more freely after that. She shared with me how much she loved her grandfather, and how he was everything to her. After that we made it back to my house. We played cards and I invited Sandy and her sister, Candy, over. They all met and hit it off cool. Monday came and I went to work, so Sonita hung out with Teric and Treyindo. By the time I got back home, they were rolling off her; everybody liked her.

She hung either over Teric's house or Treyindo's house and would come in around 1:00 in the morning.

So she wouldn't interfere with my family.

By Thursday, I had pushed up on Sandy. I knew she had an empty bedroom where she stayed and her husband wasn't coming back until March of next year. I figured by then I could have her established.

It was just Sandy and Candy's staying there with Candy two children, they had room.

Sandy said," Yeah, but you gonna have to do something for me." I said, "What?"

She said, "When the time is right, I'll tell you." I said, "bet."

I told Sonita what I had done for her and she moved in with them.

They hit it off nice. We had a New Year's Eve Party and Sonita was straight.

On her own. Susan didn't find out until later that she was there, but once she did, Susan started hanging down Sandy's house; just so she could try to cause division between them and find out information on Sonita. Sandy and Candy were shocked that Susan started coming down there on the regular so Sandy came to my job and told me. I was heated. I felt like she just didn't trust me, period!

I brought her down here and it hasn't been a good month yet before she is nick picking, just determine to find something. When I got home, I screamed on Susan. I told her," You can go back to Brooklyn if you gonna come down here with all that drama!!"

She exclaimed "Oh, did Sonita tell you that I've been coming down there?"

I said, "No!"

Then she said suspiciously "Well, it seems strange that every time I go down there she leaves and never comes back until I'm gone." I said, "She probably don't want to be bothered with you, because she knows you really don't like her!" Her eyes got big then she said, "Did she tell you that?" I twisted up my face and said,

"No, but it's obvious, so stay your ass home and watch the children, clean the house and cook me some fucking food!

You shouldn't be down there in the first place, you don't even like Sandy or Candy."

After that conversation she started cooking dinner.

There was a knock at the door and Teric and Sonita walked in.

They wanted some weed. So I gave them some. They chilled for awhile then they left.

Meanwhile, as days passed, the whole neighborhood wanted Sonita.

Sandy and Candy started looking at that as a good thing. That meant the guys would be coming over to their house and they could get on themselves. However, Sonita wasn't feeling none of the guys. Sonita would invite the guys over, leave and walk all the way to my job just to be with me. I was shocked because it was a 45- minute walk, easy. I really started liking her a lot. But, I didn't want it to seem like I was interested in her that way. I wanted to prove to her that my intentions are good and the help that she needed would come from me, out of love and concern for her; and not out of lust.

Sonita was very attractive and thorough. She wasn't scared of Susan and that really made me fond of her. Susan did a great job in intimidating everyone else, but it didn't work on Sonita.

We would walk over to the beach, to talk and play.

I felt alive again. I'll get her something to eat, then she would hop on the bus and go back home. The more she stayed around, the more Susan tried to go down to the house. However, Susan would leave around the time I was getting off from work.

I would go straight to Sandy's house so I could catch her, but she would already be gone.

Sonita would tell me the truth, but Sandy would lie for Susan. I told Sonita," listen, in one more month, Sandy's husband is going to be back, so we got to get you another place to stay." Sonita said,

"Well, let me sell some weed and I'll save my dough up and get one of these fiends to get me a spot." I said," Cool, how much can you handle?" She said, "Whatever."

So I gave her some weed to sell. It worked out for two weeks, then she and Teric (who was her hustling partner) started smoking more than what they was selling; so I cancelled that idea and just gave them enough so they could buy them some kicks, food and stay high. We laughed about it later that month, but it wasn't funny to me then.

While she was hustling though, she met this white girl named Alicea. They became real cool but I could tell Alicea was jealous of her. One day I told Sonita, and she didn't believe me, but she said that she would watch herself around her, then she hugged me and we kissed for the first time. Chills went through my whole body. I had the kool aid smile from ear to ear. Then, I walked home. At that moment, I made up in my mind that I'm going to leave Susan for her.

Little did I know, Susan already had plans on leaving me and being with somebody else.

Sonita ended up leaving Sandy's house and moved in with Alicea. They were living with this old man named Pop. He was a cool old man, all he wanted to do was drink and smoke a little weed.

Sonita used to boost beer out of Seven Eleven everyday and I supplied her with all the weed she wanted, so they was straight.

Meanwhile Susan met some people and she started smoking Crack, but I didn't know. It seemed like every time I came home; her ass was tired, the house was messed up, no food was done and the children were hungry.

I moved down the street from Sandy into a three-bedroom, so my children could have space.

I would get my cousin Jazz's car, pick Sonita up and we would go riding everywhere! I promised Sonita then that I'm leaving Susan, get an apartment for us, and we are going to be together. Sonita was very happy when I told her that. Then she said, "What about your children?" I said," they are going with me!!!!" After that I drop her off.

That night I had a very bad dream about Sonita.

She had gotten set up by the white girl Alicea, they shot her and she was in the hospital. I woke up crying real hard. Susan asked me what I was dreaming about? I told her, "About my father and how he died." She consoled me and held me. But I knew I had to see Sonita and tell her.

I couldn't find her the next day. But the following day I did. I told her, "Listen get out of Pop's house. I had a terrible dream about Alicea getting you shot and you were in the hospital." With a strange look she said,

"Are you serious?" I said,

"Yes. I don't care where you go, just go!" She said, "Alright."

That night everything was cool. However, the following night at 2:00 am someone was banging on my door.

I asked, "Who is it?" The voice said "Sonita, in a crying tone." I opened the door and she was standing there with blood all over her shirt. Her hand was wrap up in a t-shirt, but blood was pouring through it. I screamed "What the fuck happen!! Who did this to you?" She said, "You were right, Alicea got two big girls to jump me because she lied to them and said I wanted their man. I managed to get my blade out and I sliced all three of them up real bad. In the process of cutting the last girl, I cut my hand apart."

She showed me and I could see her thumb was disconnected from the rest of her fingers.

In the meantime, Susan came downstairs and caught the tail end of the story.

She said,

"You need to go to the hospital." Sonita looked at Susan and said,

"But I can't, I'm a fugitive plus the ambulance just left taking all three of them to the hospital on stretchers. They told the police who I was."

I said, "Fuck that you're going anyway!"

Susan said, "Your ass ain't going with her!" I shouted,

"I got to, she don't have nobody else.!!!"

Susan said, "I don't give a fuck. Sonita you got to go, I'm sorry but you got to leave."

So she left. I felt so bad because I couldn't do nothing.

Then I said, "Fuck that!" I got dressed and went outside looking for her.

I spotted her some ways and I called her name. She turned around crying, while she was looking at me. I said, "Here is $100.00 dollars catch a cab to the hospital and give them a fake name. I'm sorry I can't go with you. I'm going to leave this bitch. But I can't do it right now." She said,

"I understand, she's your wife. I love you Hakeem."

"I said, "I love you too." Then, I heard Susan calling me, "Hakeem! Hakeem!" I said, Bye and walked away. I hollered out, "I'm right here; stop yelling out my name!!!"

Susan said, "I fucking can't believe you! You gonna run out the fucking house for that little bitch! You gonna leave me, your fucking wife for her.?" I said, "I just wanted to make sure she was alright . I'm sorry, Susan, it wont happen again.

I hugged Susan and walked in the house.

Susan was very up set with me. I guess for the first time she actually felt that I really cared for Sonita no matter how the circumstances were between us.

The next day I was at work and Sonita called me and said, "I got stitches in my hand but I'm alright. I want you to get my clothes from Pop house for me."

I did. Alicea was putting out the word that she was gonna beat Sonita up, but everyone knew Alicea couldn't beat Sonita. Everyone was talking about how Sonita beat all three of them, at the same time. She moved in with some guy she met down the block from me. I never met him before. I asked her if she was alright there and she said yes, so I didn't pursue it any further.

Meanwhile, my wife gets a job, and after a month of laying low Sonita decides to go to Maryland with her cousin Billy. Now it's just my wife, my children and me.

Sandy's husband comes back and we all meet. Things were cool between us and we never had any problems. I met this girl who babysits.

Susan and I got her to watch our children. The girl had the most sexiest body I had ever seen.

It seemed like every time I went to pick up my children, she always had on some biker shorts or some tight spandex that hugged her body. I kept it moving, plus I met her baby's daddy.

Little did I know that he and my wife were getting high together.

Every time I came home from work, he seemed to be always just leaving the block in front of my house. I really thought nothing of it because that's where they sold their drugs. In that area. I figured he probably just got finished picking up. His girl peeped it and told me. So I confronted Susan and she denied it. But the girl wasn't having it, so she stopped babysitting our children. She wanted to fuck me to get back at him. I really didn't care what reason she used to give it up, I was with it; however it never manifested.

Mean while, one day I came home early and my children told me that when I leave to go to work, mommy would stay down the street until I came home. Then, she locks herself in the room and a funny smell starts coming out of the room. So I go upstairs and I smell Crack as I get close to the bedroom. I bust the door open and Susan is smoking Crack in her cigarette.

I snap and whipped her ass! I told her," You're going back to New York. You are not going to be down here embarrassing our children and me by your actions.

Now give me the rent money."

She started crying. I said, "What are you crying for, give me the rent money." She sobbed, "I spent it."

I said, "What? She repeated it in a low tone.

I whipped her ass some more.

She was screaming, the children were crying, but I wouldn't stop. Then I said, "Give me the rest of the food stamps we got left."

She put her head down and ran to the front door. I caught her and said, "Susan you smoked up all our money.? Where is your paycheck?"

She handed it to me, it was for $89.00. I flipped!" I yelled, "How can your check be for this much, when you leave this house everyday to go to work?" She trembled and said,

"I wasn't going to work, I was getting high. They had fired me a week ago and I was pretending like I still had the job." I dumbly said,

"I can't believe this; it's over between us, go back to New York and get some help."

I drag her to the payphone and made her call her mother and sisters to tell them what she is doing. Hopefully, they can send for her and get her some help, she refused to go.

That night I slept on the couch.

At 4:00 am Susan came creeping down the step. I'm playing like I'm asleep, but I'm watching her. She comes over to check me, then she creeps into the kitchen and stands up on the sink; she was reaching for my nine. I put it up there in case of an emergency.

However, she didn't know I had already moved it once we came in from talking to her family. When she realized it wasn't there and she turn around to get down, I smacked her to the ground. I said," Bitch you're gonna shoot me now!

Who will be here to take care of the children? huh huh?? You hate me that much that you want to kill me? You the one on drugs fucking the family all up and you want to shoot me? "

She just cried and screamed," I'm sorry I'm so sorry, I wasn't thinking."

That scared the hell out of me. I couldn't believe she hated me that much that she wanted me dead.

I told her she had to leave. She left and moved in with some girl I didn't know.

I had to find me a babysitter for my children because Susan couldn't do it.

Susan got herself a boyfriend who I never saw, and she stayed high all the time.

A week later my lights were cut off. I was mad! I figured Susan would at least pay the light bill.

When I called up the company, they told me that it was requested to be cut off by Susan Perry.

Right then I knew it was no hope for us. Anytime you would cut the lights off on your own family, you got some serious problems.

Now we were in the dark. I called Samad and told him what was going on.

He came over and suggested I move. I started looking for another place to live. In the meantime, I was taking all my children to work. They were very manageable, but they were also uncomfortable there.

It was hard for them to do their homework. I met this white girl named Tammy and she volunteered to watch my children. I really appreciated that. Now, I would drop them off at her hotel room. It was right down the street from my job, so I was able to check in on them on the regular.

Meanwhile, Susan would come up to my job and start shit every day. The only way she would leave, if I gave her $10.00 or called the cops. She really had me stressed out during this period.

Somehow she found out that I had a white girl babysitting our children. So she combed the streets trying to find her. By then, I had Tammy watching the children at our apartment. I got home early, and paid Tammy and she left to go to her place. Susan caught her, beat her up and stripped her of her clothes. The girl was terrified. Once I found out what happened, days later, I went looking for Susan to whip her ass. I couldn't find her anywhere. Tammy stop watching my kids, so I had to find someone else. That was hard because no girls around were trying to get involved with the drama. I was back to taking the kids up to my job.

I was still looking for a place because we were evicted from our apartment.

I lucked up and found a place in Mission College Apartments. The only problem was, I couldn't move in until December 9, 1995, and it's November 8th. Samad told me that we could stay with him for a week while his baby's mom was in Jamaica.

I did that and still had to have the kids with me up at the shop. When we left we would go to Samad's house. I met another girl during this period named April.

She was real cool and cute. She was from New York and we clicked really quick.

She peeped out my situation and offered to watch my kids while I work. I thanked her for it, but I had to school her on how crazy my wife was. She still did it. My brother Khalif was down in the Navy and he started coming to see me on the regular. We would go out and have fun that help me out a lot because I was really stressing.

Meanwhile, my week was up at Samad's house and April offered for us to stay with her until I could move in my place. I did. She had a daughter who was around Naquasha's age, so my kids got along good with her daughter. My kids liked April a lot. One day Susan went up to the school and the kids ran from her. She was mad!

When she finally got to talk to them, they told her that daddy got a girl friend named April and they like her. Susan was furious. She found out where we were staying and left a note in the door for April telling her that she would kill her if she continued to let us stay there. We had to move again after being there for two weeks.

I didn't have no where else to turn.

Then, my friend's mom told me we could stay there for the last week I needed before I could move into my place.

That was all I needed. However, the drama still didn't stop. After five days of being there, Susan and her girlfriend jumped Teric's mom, broke her finger, fractured her jaw, and then took the kids. I called the police and they didn't do nothing. So I went to where Susan was staying and got my children back. I felt so bad because of what happened.

I wanted to kick her ass so bad I used to dream about it. I started thinking real hard and said to my self, "This girl can't have a boyfriend because she spends everyday of her life trying to make my life miserable.

If she did' she would be with him and he wouldn't be having her following me everywhere."

Then it pop up in my mind,

That girl she is always with is her girlfriend. This chick done went gay!

FOUR
Reunited

I confronted her one day and she said, "Yes, I'm Gay." I knew it, so I wasn't even surprised. From then on I was never dealing with her again in life.

September 5,1995 was the last time we dealt and I was sticking to that until I die.

It was time for me to move in my new place.

I was $150.00 short. Bro Cooke gave me the money and told me, "Randell, just continue to serve Jehovah God." I was so happy for that. I thanked Jehovah and I brought my children to their new home. They went crazy! They ran and jumped and played all night. We had fun. I got a three- bedroom apartment with two bathrooms.

The boys had their own room and so did my daughter. They felt free and happy.

This was one of the greatest feelings I ever had; to see my children at peace.

It was our world and we were happy to be alone together.

New Year's day came and we partied. Things were peace. Khalif came around more and we were a big, happy family. Women used to bug out when they came over and it was just Khalif and me with my children. They had a lot of respect for us.

One day I get a call at the barbershop. It was Sonita! I was so shock and happy to hear from her. She said,

"Hakeem, Guess what? I stop smoking and drinking!" I said,

"Are you serious?" She proudly said,

"Yes, and I'm now in the program. I will be free in July of this year.

I had fun at my cousin Billy's house, plus I dealt with the case VA had against me.

It's all good now, Hakeem; I want to see you baby, real bad."

I was blushing on the phone. I told her, "Susan and I broke up. I have my own apartment now, so when you are finished, you can move in with me." She was thrilled about that. She said," I miss you so much, I couldn't wait to call you.

They have me staying in Sulfolk.

Our supervisors are taking us to the bowling alley in Norfolk the following week.

I want you to meet me there." I said, "Bet."

She continued, "I'm working at Burger King and I'm getting myself together." I said,

"That's great Sonita, you go girl, I knew you could do it." A customer walked in, so I told her, "I got to go baby, my client just walked in. Don't be a stranger, please call me from now on okay?" She laughed and said, "Okay." Then we hung up.

I was hype for the rest of the day.

I was very proud of her and happy things worked out for her as well.

The next week she called me and told me they were leaving to go.

I told her, "I'll be there."

I got my boy Reggie to drop me off and I walked up into the bowling alley and spotted her from the door.

She put on weight and it looked real good on her.

We hugged and kissed. She introduced me to the staff and the other girls that were in the program. We played Ms. Pac Man together. It was fun. Sonita knows I'm very competitive so we were trash talking each other. She said, "You aint nice, you used to dust me off, but who is winning now! (smile)

I said, you're not winning by much watch I beat you!" She replied, "Let's bet."

I said, "It's on, you got a deal." I was on my last man and I beat her score, then I got out.

I said "what now? You only got one more man, I'll double the bet. You won't top that."

She spoke very optimistically "Watch this!" Sonita blew pass my score and won. Afterward, we went into the lobby and talked about everything. I said,

"You know I'm waiting for you; so when you finish, you can live with me." She said,

"I wouldn't mind, but I want my own; I'm tired of living with people. If it don't work out, you know you got me." I said,

"Bet. Whatever you want to do, I will support you 100%.

Before we knew it, it was time for them to leave.

Her eyes became watery and mine did too.

We hugged, cried, kissed and said goodbye.

I didn't know how I was getting home. While I waved bye as they pulled off, this kid I knew from school was pulling out of the parking lot. He hollered,

"You need a ride?" I said, "Yes."

I got in with him and went home. I talked about her the whole way home. I loved her then, and I wanted to be with her forever.

I continued to work and take care of my children.

While their mother kept wilding the whole time.

Sonita called me every weekend. She started working full time at Burger King.

She was so focused on her goals; to finish the program and get her own on her birthday.

February rolled around and I was tired of letting my children stay with their mother on the weekend because every time they came back, they were sick. It would take me two weeks to get them better. I told Susan one night, "I'm not letting the children go with you no more. If you want to see them you're gonna have to spend time with them here."

She was mad! Susan started raising hell right in front of my apartment. I told her to calm down but she wanted the children to go with her. She was drunk and high and basically showing out for her girlfriend who was with her.

I told her to leave, it was 12:00 am.

She left. Then, in about 10 minutes later, the police are at my door with her.

I said, "What's the problem officers? They said, "This woman said you won't allow her children to leave with her." I explain to them the situation. Susan kept trying to cut me off while I was talking, so the cops made her shut up. He said,

"Well it is too late for you to be picking up some children."

I said, "That's right." But she was determined to get her way. She told them, "Well ask the children."

I said, "No they are asleep."

The cops started seeing for themselves that she wanted to just start shit.

So they ask us, "Who has custody of the children?" I said, "I do."

She said, "He is lying!"

The cop said, "Do you have proof?" I said, "Yes."

Once I showed them the papers, she was super mad.

She screamed "When did you do that?!! No body told me!" I said,

"That's because you don't have a valid address where you can be served."

She had to leave. The children were happy and they thanked me because they didn't want to go with her.

Three days later, a lady from Child Protective Services came to my place.

She said, "It's been a claim put in about me abusing my kids, as well as starving them, and she has been sent here to investigate." I said, "You can't be serious?"

I let her in and introduced her to my kids.

My kids were playing games and having a ball. I showed her their rooms, which were clean, and I showed her the refrigerator which was packed with food.

She apologized for coming by and saw for herself that these allegations were false.

She told me who made the claims, which I already knew.

For the next month, Susan and me were going to court for our children.

Finally, physical custody was granted to me, and joint custody was granted to both of us. Susan was mad about that.

However, I kept it moving. Sonita came by to visit me and my heart melted. I had butterflies in my stomach as she inspected my place. Her supervisor drops her off for a couple of hours, so we got something to eat and chilled in my place. She said," I like you're knew place. You know in July I will be finish. I want to spend my birthday with you." I said, "Thank you Sonita, and you got that. I don't mind being with you on you're birthday." She continued, "I want to let you know, I appreciate everything you done for me since we met. You have been the realest man I ever known. That's why I kept in contact with you. I'm happy you have your own, and I can't wait to be with you." I said, "I'm glad you didn't forget about me and moved on to someone else."

Sonita was looking so good with her polo shirt and blue wrangler jeans on. I wanted her so bad, but she wanted to wait until she finished the program. I respected that. We just continued to enjoy each other company until the supervisor came back to pick her up.

After that, Khalif moved in with me and we were planning to go back home to see our brothers.

We did and it was the first time all of us were together after our father died.

We put together a plan where we could make a power move and get some real dough together.

The plan was to go down in June of 96. However, once Khalif and me went up for the move, everyone wasn't ready and things went wrong.

I was mad as hell because I took my rent money to invest in this move and it fell.

I ended up losing my apartment, and my children and me were homeless.

It was all my fault.

I put more trust in my brothers instead of thinking rationally. I should know not to ever put my headrest in jeopardy. It was a lesson I will never forget. I end up moving back in with Teriq's mother temporarily, until I got me a place. It was only with the grace of God that I found a place after two weeks of living with Gwyn.

I moved to 2715 Omahundro ave in Norfolk a two bedroom apartment. Susan didn't know where I lived so it was peaceful for us. I told Sonita about my move and she said she would come see me once she got a break from her job.

Meanwhile, one night I went out to get me some beer. I had Gwyn's boyfriend watching my children. Then, when I got back, my cousin Shereef was at my place.

I was shocked. I asked him how he knew where I lived? I was only living there for a month! He told me he got the address from my brother, Ibn and caught the bus from Jersey to here; then he told the cab driver to take him to my address. I was so happy he came to see me. We are two months apart and we grew up from scratch together.

He was much taller and bigger than me.

The two of us together were unstoppable on the basketball courts, unbeatable in fights, and untouchable by the law. We did everything together. He told me he wanted to stay with me because he was on the run. I told him "No doubt it's on."

He got a job in two days. I went to the same agency and got work, now we were working together.

I felt so good to have my cousin with me. I told him all about Sonita and how she may be moving in with me. He started saving his money; in case she did come to stay, he could snatch him a place.

I was going to the Kingdom Hall of Jehovah Witnesses and was making good progress and everything, then Susan found out where I lived. But once she found out Shereef was living with me, she stopped wilding out.

Time went fast now that I had family with me. Then, one night I get a knock at my door. I ask, "Who is it?" It was Sonita! My heart jumped. I opened the door and she was standing there looking beautiful. She had on a dress. Her hair was in mini braids that were reaching down her back. I was mesmerized. This was the first time that I ever saw her in a dress.

She looked like an angel. I asked her how did she get here?

She said that her brother Eric brought her. I introduced her to Shereef. He said,

"I heard a lot about you." She said, "I hope it was good things." (smile)

Shereef replied," oh yes, very good things."

I was just blushing away. I told her, "Let me show you around." She said, "Okay."

I walked her into my room. Once we got inside, I hugged and kissed her firmly.

I told her, "I'm so happy to see you, and you look good!" She said,

"Thank you Hakeem, how have you been?" I said, "Fine, I'm just fine."

She checked my spot out and chilled for about a hour. The kids loved her and had her in their room looking at their toys. She told me she had to go and she will come see me in about two weeks. I walked her out and met her brother, then they left.

I talked Shereef to sleep about her that night.

Two weeks later she came back and told me the apartment thing didn't work out, and she had plans on moving to California with her uncle's baby mother. I was hurt.

I said, "I thought you were going to stay with me?" She said,

"You really want me to?"

I said, "Yes! Look Sonita, I got to go to this book study tonight. Would you mind waiting here until I get back? It's only for one hour?" She replied,

"Yes, Hakeem, I'll stay."

The next morning I got my friend Keith to take us to the place she was staying, so she could get her clothes. It was on from there. Shereef got him a room in this nice house on 34th Street.

He was straight. Sonita was a great help for me. She came in rearranging the house, giving it a woman's appeal. Our home looked and felt pleasant. My children always looked forward to coming home so they could be with her, and if Shereef got off early he would check on her while I was at work. We were so happy together.

On the weekends we would go out and have a ball.

Shereef would baby-sit for us and it was a very peaceful time. She became curious about the Jehovah Witnesses ever since her aunts told her not to talk to them or get away from the door. She felt like, what's wrong with them? They seem like ordinary people, just like everyone else. I set it up for her to meet Sister Young. They started studying the bible together and Sonita was so amazed at finally getting the answer to her questions that troubled her about life.

She realized what her family was telling her about the Jehovah Witnesses were lies.

The Witnesses were the only people who could answer her questions straight from out of the Bible.

Sonita had such a big heart and a great smile that lit up the room. She would tell me things about her past that really bothered her. She was really hurt and confused because her father was never in her life when he could've been. It made her feel like something was wrong with her.

However, I would always assure her that she was a beautiful person and whatever the circumstance was, she wasn't the blame.

I felt bad for her because my mother was still alive and my father was there in our lives, until he died. She lost her mother when she was 6 and met her father when she was 14. Her aunts used to tell her that her father lived down the block from her, but he never came to see her.

Sonita got in contact with her family and let them know where she was. However, not one came to visit her except her cousin Me Me and her Aunt Doreen.

Susan came over and was shocked to see Sonita at my place.

Susan ask me, "Is she your girl?" I said,

"Yes, she is. And you got the nerve to even ask me when you are fucking with girls!"

Susan was upset, but she didn't dare approach Sonita. She left.

The next day while my kids, Sonita and I were at Granby Park, I proposed to Sonita. She smiled and said, "Yes."

I gave her the engagement ring I bought.

That night we cooked a big dinner, ate and played music.

My children were dancing and singing songs. We danced and sang along.

Sonita was so happy, she cried after the children went to bed.

I asked her, "What was wrong?"

Sonita said, "All I ever wanted was to be loved and be with my family.

Since my mom passed my family has never been there as a whole.

I admire your relationship with your children. I'm happy that they love and accept me."

I told her, "All I ever wanted was a woman I could love and give my all too.

Sonita, I'm happy you allowed me to be with you." I wiped the tears from her eyes and kissed her. As we got passionate with each other, I picked her up and laid her in the bed.

We immediately began to take each other clothes off, and I wasted no time burying my face into her luscious pussy.

She held a firm grip on my head as I sucked out all her juices.

Her body began to tremble, but I wouldn't let up on pleasing her. Finally, I plunged my dick deep in her tight pussy and she dug her nails into my back, while I pound away into her sexy body.

We made love the whole night. However, something strange kept happening.

Every time we do it and she felt good, she would stop and go to the bathroom, but each time she came back, she'd say, "I didn't have to use it."

She didn't understand why. So I asked her," You know woman can come too right?"

She said, "No, how?"

I said, "You never came before?" She said,

"No, but I do get this feeling like I got to pee, but it never happen when I go in the bathroom."

I chuckled inside. Then, I explained to her, when you get that feeling you don't stop, just pee; and I guarantee baby, you will climax and have an orgasm.

When we did it again and she came she screamed like crazy!

Afterwards, she said, "Give me that feeling again!

It was an experience we both couldn't get enough of.

Sonita learned the completion to making love and the loyalty of a man who would give his all. She was satisfied and complete. She got a job at Farm Fresh down the block from the house.

We were balling from that point all. However, Susan did her best to complicate matters and Sonita end up moving in with Me Me. I ended up losing my apartment, so I went to a shelter.

While I was there, Sonita came to visit me from V.A. Whenever her schedule would allow.

During that time, I was in the midst of changing jobs. I end up at Jed Shop on Colley Avenue. Spoon helped me get in there and it worked out fine for me.

The only problem I had was having a babysitter to watch my kids while I was at work.

Some ladies in the facility volunteered but, they wanted me to fuck them for their services.

One of them would have gotten it, but I didn't pursue it.

I knew I had Sonita as my girl so I was straight on being intimate.

I paid the woman who watched my kids and that was it. In the meantime all the woman used to come to my room and talk.

The conversations were peaceful and we all were able to get a good night's sleep. When Ms Mosley walk through and gave her count, she noticed me writing in my notebook.

One day she asked me, "What are you writing?" I said, "My book." She asked,
"What's your book about?"
I said, "My life."
She said, "Let me read it."
I did. I only had about 7 chapters done, but I let her read it.
A couple of days passed and Ms Letriece Mosley came in to work.
The first thing she asked me was, is my book true?
"I said, "Yes."
She later called my mom to find out if what I wrote was true, without my knowledge.

Ms Letriece Mosley was very impressed with my book, and she offered to help me get it published once I finished it. I felt good about that because here is a stranger, who read just a couple of chapters and was willing to lend a helping hand. I was very grateful.

Finally, I told her about the songs I have and she listened to me.

Our conversations were so healthy and uplifting to me that I really didn't feel ashamed or bad about living in the shelter. I realized then it's just a period in my life that, I'm going through. To be successful comes from hitting rock bottom, and coming up strong, radiant, and bright.

Ms Letriece told me about her son Timberland.

At the time, I didn't have the slightest idea who he was.

She told me about his two encounters with death, and how loving and blessed he is.

Timberland and his brother were her whole life. It really got amazing during them times because I looked at her as my mother who was not there for me, because of the distance. Ms Letriece showed me unconditional love and she also fell in love with my two sons Randell Jr a.k.a. Love and Rahshon, who we nicknamed Rah Diggidy.

I ended up telling Ms Letriece my life and she told me hers, especially about her fiancé' she was about to marry, plus the great relationship she has with her two sons.

As we got deeper with our history, I found out she knew Sonita's mother and her whole family.

Sonita's aunt was her best friend. That alone cemented my love and devotion to her.

Sonita did the whole 45- days stay with me. Unfortunately my cousin Shereef died in Jersey just three weeks after he left V.A. to be with this girl he was in love with.

He moved to Atlanta with her and things didn't work out, so he went back to Jersey and died.

My brother Ibn was doing good at that time and he vowed to give me whatever I needed to come home. I told Sonita that I loved her; however, I was moving back home.

She immediately said, "I'm going with you."

"I said, "Word! You are willing to go to Jersey with me?"

"She said, "You damn right!"

I said, "It's on then."

FIVE
Jersey Bound

My friend Jed, who was my boss at the time, gave me his condolence in regards my cousin passing.

He let me cut in the shop for free so I could have money to travel with.

Spoon encouraged me to be strong.

Sonita told her grandfather she was moving to New Jersey with me and he didn't want her to go.

He thought I'd probably dog her out or kill her, but she knew better and she bounced with me.

Her brother Eric dropped her off to me , and we had a nice, long conversation. I could tell he was concern about his little sister.

He asked me, "Promise me you will take good care of my sister." I said,

"Oh, no doubt, I love your sister; she is my heart." We shook hands and he left.

This day was very hectic, I didn't have no license or no way of renting a Uhaul Truck to drive to New Jersey. Being that I did good while at the shelter, they gave me everything I needed for my apartment. I felt like crying for real because I couldn't believe how nice these people were. After they walked me through everything that I could have, I had to find someone to rent a Uhaul truck for me. Sonita suggested I ask Jed or Spoon, but I felt like they had done enough.

Then she said, "We'll what about Indoe?"

I said, "Word! Let's go past 36 St and see if he,s home."

We went and he was there. We asked him and he said yeah. We got the U-haul Truck and loaded it up with my furniture. Brand new living room set, kitchen set, bedroom set two, 9 foot mirrors, entertainment center, a TV, two vcrs, all of our clothes and belongings.

My money was tight, so I gave Indoe one of the vcrs. He was straight.

We got on the road at 7:00pm. Sonita, Randell jr, Rahshon and me.

This was the first time that I was driving to New Jersey, because all the other times I was on the bus.

It was April 1,1997. I didn't let my nervousness show around Sonita because she was very hyped on the ride. This was the first time she was leaving V.A. to go live in New Jersey.

Her happy, optimistic spirit kept me up. I was so happy to know that she loved and trusted me that much to go to my hometown. Randell Jr. and Rahshon were knocked out sleep.

Sonita did her best to hang out with me, however, by the time we reach Jersey she was out sleep. We arrive there around 2:00am. I introduced Sonita to my grandmother.

They clicked from the door. I was shocked because I knew my grandma really wasn't too fond of me. However, she took to Sonita quick.

That morning she met Dawu and Ibn.

We had fun and she was very happy.

For one, she was out of V.A. and for two she was with the man whom she loved.

Everybody on my mother's side of the family came by to see us for the next couple of days.

I took Sonita to my mother so they could meet. Sonita was so scared; however, I assured her my mom was cool. They met and I left Sonita with my mom for about an hour while I walked the streets of Newark looking for people I knew. I ran into my brother Kasseem and he walked back with me to my mother's place. Sonita was having a good time. She and my mom got along great.

My mom gave us her blessings and we left from there and went to see Yolanda and Charmaine, (Shereef's sisters,) Ronnie was with us.

Sonita was nervous because we had to go to the projects.

Our projects were totally different from what she knew. She had never been in a building 30 stories high. The elevator was messed up so we had to walk up 15 flights of stairs, encountering all kinds of people as we climbed; crack heads, stick up kids, car thieves, drug dealers, and killers. She held my hand very tight. She met Charmaine. Charmaine told me what happened with Shereef it had me in tears. Shereef was my closest first cousin. We were only two months apart. I was devastated.

We left from the projects and went back to my grandmother's house.

The funeral was on my birthday, April 5,1997.

I didn't know how I was going to get there. I didn't have a ride, but I had my family.

I began to have nightmares every night.

All that kept running through my head was our last conversation.

I practically begged him not to leave with this girl. He was doing so good. Shereef found a job in two days after being in V.A.; months later he had his own place, and in three more weeks he was about to get a ride. He also started reading the Bible again.

He told me how proud he was that I was serving Jehovah God.

We used to talk about our life at lunchtime on top of the building we were renovating.

Now he was gone! I'm confused, hurt, mad, shocked, in denial, and don't know what to do.

As the day turned out, it was only God's doing that allowed me to use my brother Ibn's Green Range Rover to go to the funeral with my family. It was comfortable.

I was trippin' because I was under the pretense that his girlfriend in Atlanta food poisoned him. So, when I saw her there, I wanted to beat her up. When I started to go towards her, Yolanda told me not to because she was going to take care of her.

Nonetheless, it did nothing towards calming me down. I was so mad, upset, and confused because my best and first cousin was dead for no apparent reason.

It was tough, but we managed to move on. As the months passed 15 more friends and family members of mine died and Sonita felt emotionally disturb with that. Never before in her life had she seen so much death.

Every other person she had met through me died.

It was a big strain on our relationship because my family hadn't seen me in three years and they were coming to see me in bunches.

Each time they came unannounced or invited Sonita didn't like it.

She felt neglected and upset with my family taking up all our time. I tried to help her understand that I'm the cornerstone and backbone to the family, I'm the only one everybody gets along with.

It wasn't like when they came I left and came back home in the late hours of the night.

They seemed to stay at our house too long for her.

Her beef was, when is she going to have her time with her man?

If I did go out, she would be terrified that I wouldn't be coming back home.

She felt I would be next to die and that stressed her out. I was all she had.

I'm ignorant to the fact and think she's just trippin'.

In the meantime, she got a job at this diner in Irvington.

She only worked a week before she found a better job at Pep Boys, dealing with fixing cars. However, she met some girl at the diner who became fond of her. To Sonita, she seem like a cool, fun girl. Personally, I can see she was a dike. And I didn't like her.

Anyway, she came around from time to time to see Sonita.

I was cool with it long as they never left my house.

But the girl would always invite Sonita to go with her places.

Sonita had love and respect for me, so she would ask me if it was cool.

I told her no. She was mad because she felt she had to be confined to the house.

I understood how she felt, however I knew in my heart that I couldn't let anything happen to her up here in New Jersey.

I wouldn't be able to face myself or her family.

In the meantime though, she busted the job out at Pep Boys, and everybody was sweating her.

She saw the splendor of Jersey's finest men. They stayed on her heels to the point she told me about her stalkers and one dude who was offering her $20,000.00 to marry his son from another country.

I felt like the dude from Indecent Proposal; however the love of my life wasn't marrying no one but me! We had so much fun in the mist of all the drama that was going on around us; until this girl comes over to the house on her day off trying to get her to go to New York with her. Now, I took it personal. There was no way this dike girl is going to take my girl, who I promised back in V.A., to the Big Apple.

However, I didn't say that to Sonita; I told her no!

She was mad, so she punched me in the mouth and busted my lip.

Then, she started screaming, "I don't do nothing but work and stay in the house, I want to go out and you won't let me leave with the only friend I got!! Why, I can handle myself!" I said,

"I know you can baby, but the point is, I don't know her, where she lives, or if she is who she claim. You met a lot of my female cousins and friends and I never deprived you from going out with them?" She shouted,

"I don't care about your people; this is someone I met on my own and I trust her enough to go out with her." I replied with,

"We'll, it ain't happening, so you might as well punch me in my shit again, because you are not leaving."

Randell Jr. and Rahdiggidy were right there on the couch as I stood in the doorway bleeding from my mouth.

She looked at my kids, then back at me and went to the window to tell the girl she wasn't going.

The girl was mad and just spun out in her car. I made dinner and fed the family.

After the boys went to sleep, we talked about our differences, made up, then we made love.

Two weeks later was the fourth of July. She had the day off from work and so did I.

I'm trying to enjoy the fireworks outside and get a breather from Sonita because she kept telling me something was wrong with her.

I figured she just wanted more of my attention.

Little did I know something was really bothering her.

Anyway, I'm ignoring her on the porch.

She's in the window telling me to come upstairs right now! I said, "No, wait until I finish my forty and see the fireworks."

She slammed the window down and went into the kitchen.

I finished half of my forty and peeped half of the fireworks, then went upstairs.

She locked me out. I had to kick the door to get in.

She opened the door and said, "You don't fucking love me!"

I said, "Your buggin'" while I stumbled in the house. She said, "Fuck you and threw bleach all over me. Some of it went in my eyes and they burned like hell.

I charged her and took the bleach from her.

I poured the rest of my beer on her and she flipped. She started fighting.

I didn't want to hit her because she is the girl I love. It's not in my nature to fight woman, but she stabbed me twice in front of my sons. They are screaming because they are scared. I'm bleeding from my chest and arms. Anyhow, I hit her once. She fell and started screaming," You hit me, you hit me!" I said,

"Sonita, you made me do it; why? I fucking love you girl." Then she said,

"No, you don't because you never listen to me, or care about my feelings."

We both cried in each others arms; then she got dressed. I said, "Where are you going?"

She said, "Out." I didn't stop her. Thirty minutes later, I see her walking towards the house so I go downstairs to meet her. I ask her if she was alright, then I apologized.

She said she was fine.

Ten minutes after that, two cop cars pulled up.

First thing came to my mind was, we just got passed the fighting, now we are talking and the cops come.

She knew my heart couldn't sit well with no woman who would call the cops on me.

Then my mind said, "Fuck it." I got a good alias.

Stay humble and talk your way out of this shit.

She knows I got warrants for my arrest. We just don't know how many and for what.

But all of that went out the window because Sonita started popping shit. She yelled,

"Now motherfucker, you gonna hit me now; watch your ass go to jail!"

Three cops got out of two cars. A big, fat black cop and a slim white cop got out of the first car. They walked straight up to us. The other white cop followed slowly. I spoke humble to the cops while she was all irate. Now, they can see she's upset, but she is not in any immediate danger.

They notice two boys in the window looking puzzled.

The black cop asked if they were her children and she said, "No they are his."

They asked me my side and I basically said it was a big misunderstanding; I feel we can work it out.

She said, "No we can't because I'm leaving you!"

I was hurt by those words, but I manage to hold a smile. The cops said,

"Listen mam, we can see you're not in any immediate danger. Your boyfriend's kids are here, it's just you four. We're gonna run a check on him. If he's fine, we'll leave, and you two try to work out your differences."

I said, "Thank you officers! I appreciate that."

I knew my alias was clean and I had the I.D. to confirm that.

She said, "Okay." and then pulled out my real I.D. next, she gives it to the officers.

After that, she looked at me with the most evil look I had ever seen. I was shocked!!!

I knew it was over for me because I had violated my probation.

The police check came back with five warrants for my arrest.

I was crushed, hurt, and pissed off!

The officers felt bad for me, so the white officer asked Sonita not to press charges because I had five warrants. He said, "He's finished if you press charges."

She said, "Fuck him, lock him up!

I walked over to the white officer so he could arrest me.

The black officer said, "We'll, can you go up stairs and move the children out the window so they don't see us arresting Mr.Barkley?"

I couldn't believe how they finally got me.

I was on the run for three years, and they catch me by the hands of my girl, on a humble.

When she went upstairs the black officers said, "You know you can press charges on her? You're bleeding from your chest and your arms."

The white officer said, "We can call you an ambulance."

The third officer cut in and said,

"We got to arrest him; just take him to the hospital first.

Then the black officer said, "When she comes back down, we're gonna ask her again.

If she wants to pursue it, we're gonna lock her up too because of what she did to you; but if she won't pursue it, we'll let her walk.

I said, "Bet."

She came downstairs. By then, they had already put me in the car.

I sat there and listened to what the officers said. They were really trying to persuade her, but she was determined to add on to whatever beefs I already had.

They grabbed her and told her she was under arrest for aggravated assault with a deadly weapon. Her whole facial _expression changed. She started crying and stated that she changed her mind. However, it was too late..

In the mist of this going on, my older cousin Teric, who babysat the boys while we were at work. He just so happened to walk up.

I told the officer that he was my family and that my children can stay with him.

That way, they wouldn't have to go to the precinct until I got some one to pick them up.

I told the officer to give him my wallet so he may have money for the kids; plus change to call people. My other reason was because I knew my alias I.D. was in my wallet.

I know how the searches go down once you're in. They would have caught it and I would have another charge. They put her in the other car and took her straight to jail. They took me to the hospital so I could get treated for my injuries. Then, I arrived at the jail three hours later.

They fed me and everything. Mad jokers were locked up for Domestic Violence.

Least 20 guys, and 2 girls. One was Sonita and the other girl was in for shoplifting.

I was the only one who the cops, that night, let counter complain. When jokers saw how I was bandaged up, they thought my girl must be a beast. I knew at least half of the guys.

We were buggin' out; making the best out of it because some of us know we are going to the County or Caldwell, and we will have to prove ourselves; but for now, we are going to breathe about our situation that got us here. Sonita heard my voice through the walls and she called out to me saying she is sorry and she loves me.

I told her, "I love you too, but things are gonna change."

Then she told me that the girl who was in there with her said that Sonita was pregnant, that's why she is buggin'. I said,

"Don't believe any of these locked up fake psychics or fake doctors!"

Everyone started laughing. I really didn't mean for it to be funny; it just came out that way. The next day came and it was a Sunday. The fellas knew we were stuck until Monday before we see court.

It started getting crowded. Sonita had the C.O. give me her food because she couldn't see eating bread and cheese without any mayo or mustard.

We talked to each other, peacefully, through the walls.

I couldn't hear her totally clear, but the guys who were closer to her side could.

They would repeat what she said for me. Sunday night came and the precinct had called the judge at home so he could post bail on some of the inmates because they needed room for more people.

They called out the names of all who could go home on their own recognizance.

Sonita's name was one of them.

They announced all who would be jail drop; this was the girl, nine others, and me.

Sonita screamed out" Hakeem! Hakeem, fuck you. I'm leaving your ass!"

Brothers started laughing, cracking jokes, saying she was lovey dovey with you until she heard she could go and you got to stay.

I said," Alright fellas, don't blow it out of proportion." One hour later they started letting people go.

I couldn't see who left because of my side of the jail, however, the other guys that were left could.

When they saw Sonita, they went crazy! They were like, she look good as hell!

She can't be from here cause of how she look and talk. That pretty, small, girl cut you up like that?

I said, "Yeah, don't get it twisted, she's thorough!

Monday came and I was jail dropped to the County. I stayed there for two days.

I talked to my brother Dawu and he was steamed! He wanted to do something to Sonita, but I told him, "No, she is my girl. I'll deal with her my way."

The third day, they sent me to Caldwell. I met some cool people and I didn't have not one beef with anybody. I was comfortable, but stressed out because I didn't know what she was doing. I didn't know how my sons were and that seriously fucked me up.

I didn't have not one idea why I had four other warrants. I was thinking about all the fucked up shit I did back in New Jersey.

Thinking someone ratted me out. The young brother in my cell was thorough as hell! He was from Prince Street Projects.

He gave me an envelope so I could write her and I did, a five page letter.

She never wrote back nor went anywhere around my family. However, Ibn and Khalif patrolled my home just to make sure nothing was going on. After the first week, they started calling me to court for my beefs. Probation violation, child support, armed robbery, car jacking, assault on a minor.

I beat the child support because my kids were with me. Armed robbery and carjacking were drop because, they didn't have enough evidence to convict me for it. They reinstated my probation. Another week goes by and at 9:00pm they told me to pack my shit up. I didn't know if they were going to move me to another wing in the building, therefore, I asked the C.O. "What's up?" He said, "You're going to the County. I said, "But I rather stay here." He said, "What? You rather stay here, than go home?" I said, "They are letting me go?"

He said, "That's what's on the transcript." I was shocked.

I felt like they were making a mistake, but I damn sure wasn't going to correct it.

I went to the county with 12 others. They let all of us go except two people.

I didn't call any body or nothing. I just walked home. For two and a half weeks I'd been locked up and the word was out that I was looking at three years in prison.

Once I arrived at my place, the door was opened. The apartment was rearranged, a curtain divided the kitchen from the living room, and some furniture was missing.

As I walked through the hallway, I could hear voices, someone said, I'm a wait for you downstairs." Then I heard Sonita say alright. I rushed into the bedroom and it was a dike looking girl leaving out. She screamed, "Aaaah! Sonita some man is in your house!"

I shouted, "Bitch, this is my house, and you better get the fuck out right now!"

The girl ran passed me and I walked further into the bedroom. Sonita was putting on her shirt and fixing her pants. She was shocked to see me. I yelled at her and said," You fucking with girls now! Why don't you have on your clothes?" She said, "You know damn well I don't mess with girls Hakeem, I just got off of work. I was changing clothes because I was on my way down the block." I cut her off and said, "For what, huh. Tell me for what? Matter of fact where are my sons and who was that girl?"

She stuttered and said," Hakeem, I, I, don't want you to be mad but, To Susan got the boys. Your mother sent her to get them because I didn't have a baby sitter. I'm so sorry baby."

I just busted out in tears, I couldn't believe my sons were gone and I walked in on her getting dress in front of a dike. I screamed out, "You got my son's tooking from me, I wrote you letters and you didn't write me back or come to visit me. Since I known you, I always looked out for you, and this is the thanks I get! Who is this girl and where did you meet her?" She said, I met her through your cousin Nick, he been by to check up on me, so I would go down to her house and play cards and drink. I don't have no friends, and I couldn't go around your brothers. Hakeem I'm really sorry for what I done. I love you and I wouldn't mess with no one out here. I'm not like that. I just needed someone to talk to. Baby, take off your clothes and I'll run you some bath water and wash you up. If you don't want to be bothered with me I'll move back down south."

I said, "We'll, that's exactly where your going, because I can't seem to trust you anymore. Here I am locked up because of you and you're over niggers houses playing cards and enjoying life right!" She sobs and said, "It's not like that Hakeem, for real. I'm lost without you. Please give me one more chance." Then she started crying.

I walked into the living room and broke down again. All the memories I experienced with her and my sons were running through my head. Sonita went and ran some bath water and tried to console me. All I could think of was, my sons are gone, my girl cheated on me, and I only been gone for two and a half weeks.

I didn't believe her. I was very upset from what she told me. She said,

"Look Love, when I got your letter, I was confused because Dawu told me you were going to fuck me up.

Therefore the best thing for me to do was move. I didn't know what to believe."

I told her, "He lied because he was mad about what you did to me, plus I wouldn't give him the okay to hurt you.

He figured I was shot out over you. He wasn't trying to see me get played."

After I washed and got dressed I told her, "If you want to leave me, go ahead; I'm staying in Jersey."

I left and went to call my mother. I cursed my mother out for calling Susan and doing things behind my back.

I then went to my brother's house. They were shocked to see me, and they told me what was going on since I was gone.

Khalif said, "I did see a guy going up in your apartment around two oclock in the morning. I went up stairs and banged on the door. Sonita answer it.

When she open the door the dude was sitting on your couch. Sonita said,

"What's wrong Khalif?"

Khalif said, "What's wrong? Why the fuck is this dude up in my brother's house?"

The dude got scared and left. Khalif told her, "I don't care if my brother is locked up you ain't fucking with no body around here, and especially up in his house! She said,

"He was a friend." Khalif said, "My brother, is your only friend."

Then, he left. I was hurt and confused but I didn't let it show.

I left and went back to my house.

By the time I got back, the house was clean and Sonita was making dinner.

When she looked at me, she could clearly see something was wrong.

Sonita said, "What is it? What did your brothers tell you?" I said, "Something you didn't."

I told her and she just put her head down. Sonita said, "I know it don't look right, but I didn't fuck him. What, do you think I'm just that easy? Huh, like I don't got no morals. True, I was very lonely while you was gone, and I needed someone to talk to.

I couldn't go to your family, they all hated me for telling on you.

I was scared to death, and stressed out. I realized I didn't think it through when I got you locked up. I just wanted you to hurt like you hurt me. I'm sorry Love I really am.

I love you."

I felt she was telling me the truth at that point. She was very sincere.

However, I couldn't get past the facts. Another man was in my house, taking my family out. Once my children left he is coming over late at night.

If he didn't hit it, he was damn near on his way.

What if I was still locked up? Those thoughts plagued my mind.

I felt hopeless, stupid, and naive. There was no doubt in my mind that I still loved her.

I figured I'd make sure she gets back to V.A. safe and just live my life.

That night we made love and it felt different.

I don't know if it was my mind playing tricks on me, or my inner senses being on point.

Sonita asked me, "What's wrong?" I just started crying nonstop.

I couldn't explain to her my reason, however she said, "What, I don't feel right to you?

You really think I cheated on you? "

I said, "Yes, because I'm still shocked how you turned your back on me.

How can I put this past you?

You didn't consider me your man when they released you, plus you normally wouldn't talk to anyone."

She looked puzzled. Then she said, "You're right, I wouldn't, but I didn't know if you still loved me.

I'll prove it to you tomorrow. You can meet him and ask him yourself."

I said, "Bet."

The next day, we went to the dude's house.

When he saw her I could see his whole face light up.

He said, "Hi Sonita. Then, I walked up. He had a confused look on his face.

She introduced me as Love, her man; and then she said, "This is the guy that was willing to help me move back to V.A."

I said, "Whatever, dig. Did you fuck my girl?"

He quickly replied, "Oh no, I was just trying to help." I said,

"Save that bullshit for someone else. Did you?"

I started getting hyped. Sonita grabbed me and said, Love, he answered you baby, lets go." The dude backed up in his doorway and said, "Take it easy Sonita.

I don't want no problem. All she did was talk about you."

I said, "What!"

Sonita said, "I'm sorry, I intervened and said, "Fuck you, apologizing to this cat for what?" She said,

"Because I didn't expect you to act like this."

I said, "Fuck him!"

Then she laughed as we walked away. I said, "What's so funny?" She said,

"You were all ready to fight that guy over me. (smile). You really love me, huh?"

I looked at her and said,

"Yeah, you're my heart."

The next morning Sonita was throwing up. I asked her if she was alright? She said,

"I've been throwing up for the last week."

I said,

"Word, take some Tylenol or something." Then I left.

I came back to her 4 hours later, and she still wasn't feeling right. We went to the hospital.

I had to make a money move with my brother and the hospital was taking forever.

Sonita started stressing me out while I was there.

Eventually, I left her there.

I went and made the move with my brother and I came home later.

By then, she was just coming from the hospital.

I didn't care what was wrong now, because if it was serious they would've kept her.

Sonita said, "That's fucked up; you left me in the hospital.

I told her,

"I had to get the rent money up and staying in there wasn't going to do it."

She looked at me and said,

"Well do you want to know what the doctor said?"

Sarcastically, I said, "What." She said, "I'm pregnant." I was speechless.

My whole attitude towards her changed. Suddenly I was very happy.

She said the doctor told her that's why she's been acting so irate and throwing up in the mornings. We went into the house and I made dinner. The following day I told my brothers and Dawu said, "Well, is it yours?"

And a lightening bolt popped in my head. I've been with her for two years and she never got pregnant.

I get locked up for two and a half weeks and now she is popped up.

I went back to the house and asked her, "How many weeks are you?" She said,

"Love; what, you don't think it's yours?" She began to cry. "If you don't want the baby, I'm still having it." I said,

"It's not that. If its mine, of course I want it." She surprisingly said,

"What do you mean, if its yours. Love, I haven't been with no body else." She cried profusely and went into the room.

I felt bad. So I walked in there and tried to hold her, but she didn't want to be bothered.

I sat on the bed and apologized for what I said.

Sonita said, "Next week is my next appointment, would you go with me then we can find out together?"

We did. She was 6 weeks, which meant she got pregnant two weeks before we were locked up.

I was relieved. That explained her outbursts and her taking things to the extreme.

Now, moving back to V.A. was out of the question. We were going to stay together.

I contacted Susan in the meantime and told her I was coming to V.A. to get the children and she said, "I don't mind."

That was set up for down the road. Sonita told her family back home and they were happy for her.

This cemented our love for each other because she wanted a baby very bad.

Someone she can love and was a part of her. All the drama we took each other through went out the window. We started preparing for this new arrival.

We've been with each other since '94 now in '97 she's pregnant with our first child together.

SIX

First Born

It's the third week in August. It's hot and people are out everywhere.

I'm hustling and cutting hair out of my house.

Sonita is still working. I find out that one of my younger sisters had her first child.

I decided to go over there to see her. I told Sonita, once she came home, where I was going and I left.

I caught the cab over there and all that was on my mind was my baby sister had her first child. I'm an uncle on my mother's side.

I got out of the cab and rang the doorbell. My sister Katrina came to the door.

She smiled and I smiled and we hugged. I said, "Congratulations, sis; where is my niece?" She said,

"In my room." I said, "Word." I walked in and saw my niece for the first time.

I said to myself, Damn, that baby looks just like Bernard. I told her,

"She looks just like you, she's cute."

By then, I was expecting my mother to walk in but she didn't.

Out of curiosity, I asked Katrina "Where is mommy?"

She said, "Oh, you didn't know; she's been in the hospital for two weeks now.

She is in I.C.U. I said, "What! Why? What happened?" Ironically, while I was talking, Bernard was getting out of the bed.

He headed for the door which would take him up stairs to his parent's house.

Katrina continued, "Well, she was stressing over ya'll's last conversation and she wanted to see you; however, Bernard didn't want her too. He gave her some medicine from the hospital and it messed her up. Her stomach was bloated and she couldn't breathe. He took her to the hospital and since then she has been in I.C.U."

My head was royally fuck up!

All I could think about was the last conversation we had.

I did get smart with her, only because I felt she didn't believe in me. She told me though, "that I need to calm down and focus on Sonita because, she came from a another state to be with you, son. That's who you should stand by.

Forget your brothers, they won't be there after some real stuff happens to you."

Now my mother is in I.C.U.

I couldn't think straight. My first instinct was to run upstairs and fuck Bernard up.

Then, my next instinct was forget him go to the hospital. I asked Katrina what hospital. She said, "University."

I had her call me a cab and I was going to the hospital to see my mom!

I went in the first door.

I gave my mother's name and they gave me the floor. I went on the floor and asked for the room.

They told me the room and I walked to it. However, there was a fat, dark skinned lady in there with a bald head.

I knew from the door that wasn't my mother. Inquisitively I went to all eight rooms that were left and I still couldn't find her.

I thought they may had moved her because she is doing better.

Therefore, I asked the lady again, "Are you sure my mother is in 17, because I went in there and I didn't see her?"

The nurse said, "Yes, that is Mrs. Broughton."

I looked puzzled as hell.

Then, I walked back in the room to take a closer look, and it was my mother!

She looked like death in the purest form!

Her body was bloated, she lost her complexion, and all of her hair fell out. I started throwing up from the sight of her.

I couldn't hold it. Then, my other sister Christie came into the room. She held me and cleaned me up.

She filled me in on the law suit scandal Bernard had devised.

Some way my mother was getting money from an accident that I didn't know anything about. Bernard was hoping my mom passed before anybody could find out.

I was furious at Bernard! Death was all I could conceive for the man.

He was going to wear it. On my life!

I started talking to my mother and she responded! It shocked Christie because she has been incoherent for three days.

I asked her what happened and she told me, verbatim, about our last conversation and how Bernard gave her some medicine and it hurt her stomach.

She started tearing up when she said, "I'm sorry I look like this son." I said,

"Like what? I don't care how you look, you're my mommy."

Her lips were chapped and her teeth were yellow. I asked her,

"Do you want some Ice?" She shook her head, yes.

Christie ran out of the room to get the doctors.

When they came in, they were shocked to hear me carrying on conversation with my mother.

The doctor wanted to ask her some questions. He said,

"Who are you talking to, Mardette?" My mom said, "My son."

The doctor ask her, "Well, what is his name?" She said, "Randell!"

He looked back at the other doctor and nurses and smiled. He said, He couldn't believe it. She almost died twice since she's been in the hospital. Incoherent the whole time and now her son comes in and she is responsive! I asked the doctor,

"What's wrong with my mother?"

He said, "Let's step out in the hallway." Christie stayed inside with our mother and started feeding her ice.

The doctor said, "Your moms is in the final stage of cancer.

It's nothing we can do for her, I'm sorry."

I said, "What do you mean its nothing you can do for her? You just said she is coherent, she's probably going to come out of it."

He said, "Sir, the Cancer has spreaded through her body. You should try to prepare for her demise. I told him,

"Fuck that, she will get better and when she does I'm going to have her stay with me."

The doctor responded, "Okay sir, okay. We will do all we can." Then, he walked away.

I called him back and said. "Look doc, I'm sorry if I have been hostile towards you, I'm just hurting right now.

He said, "Sir I understand, it's hard for us to look on and not be able to do anything.

I felt the lump in my throat and the tears ready to fall, but I held it back and mustard up a smile, then I walked back into the room. Christie told me that she's been up there for the last couple of days and mommy is actually looking better than when she first came. All I could think of was mommy look terrible now, I'm in shock. I'm confused as hell; what am I going to do? Not my mom I don't have anybody left as it is. My father died June 22,1988 and here is my mom laying on her death bed in August of 1997.

I know Christie was talking to me for a minute and I was in a daze.

She grabs me and said, "Randell, do you hear me talking to you?"

I said, "Damn, sis, I'm sorry. I got to call my job." Then, I walked back out. I used the phone in the waiting room. I called my job and explained to my boss what was going on.

I then started calling all my people on my mother's side so they could know what was going on.

I left after that and went home to Sonita. She was all happy and upbeat.

She told me dinner will be ready shortly.

She was rushing a little bit just to make things nice for me. However, I told her, "You don't have to do that baby, I need to talk to you." Then when she turned around and look in my eyes, she could tell something was wrong.

She hugged me and kiss me, then asked me what was wrong?

I broke down right there and told her everything.

She just held me and let me cry in her arms. That made me feel so good because Sonita was the only woman who held qualities as my mom so I could express myself without feeling embarrassed.

She told me, "Well just go down there everyday and be with her. I'll stay here and wait for you to come home."

I told her, "Christie and I are going to do shifts with her."

Sonita told me, "That was good to do."

The next day I went, I ran into my uncle Randy.

He's my mother oldest brother.

She looked out for him all her life.

Even though he did a lot of fucked up shit to her.

I was very happy to see him here. I spoke and smiled. He told me, "I see my sister is doing bad, I feel for you Randell."

He patted me on the back. I felt like breaking down, but I held on for some reason.

As we got closer to the room, he switched his demeanor.

Then he said,

"Now look Randell, you are just Mardette's son. Bernard is her husband, so don't be trying to go against what he tells the doctors to do!"

I said, "What!" The first thing that came across my mind was the fact, I never ever stepped up to my Uncle Randy because I love and respect him. But, he just revealed to me that he was on Bernard's side, knowing this guy is the cause of my mom's problem.

I knew right then Bernard had to have given Randy some money.

I jumped right in Randy's face and told him, "Fuck you and Bernard! That's my mom and ain't no decision gonna be made without my consent."

Then he said, "But that's his wife!" I said, "Motherfucker, that's my mother and your baby sister! And I can't believe you are siding with this nigger over my mother Randy, stay the fuck out of my face! He said, "Oh, you think you tough now; you can just talk to me however you want." I looked right into Randy's eyes and said, "Stay away from me!" When I turned into the room, my Aunt Kim was in there and so was Bernard. He could see on my face that I was already steamed. He started talking to Kim, but she began hugging me, crying and I embraced her.

Randy said, "Just listen because you are hardheaded." I said, "Fuck you," calm as hell.

Then Randy said to Bernard,

"Look I'm about to leave; I'll come by the house and see you."

However, Bernard said, "No, don't leave yet; I'll go with you." He immediately walked past me and followed Randy out. I thought to myself that money had to be involved for Randy to do this. I went into the room, hugged and kissed my mother. She woke up and managed to muster up a smile. I cracked some jokes with both of them. They both started laughing.

My mother really couldn't laugh to her capacity, so she chuckled. I told my mother that Sonita was pregnant and she smiled then said,

"That's wonderful, tell her congratulations." I said, "Okay."

At that moment, my mother was filled with life.

She understood everything we were talking about.

She would either nod her head yes or no. Then, out of nowhere, my Aunt Kim told me how Bernard gave Randy $400.00 to scare me off from coming up to the hospital. Talking about how I'm causing controversy in the hospital and I'm giving the doctors a hard time. Then, he turn to her and gave her $20.00 to mind her business. She was mad as hell behind it but she took the $20.00 I couldn't blame her. Kim didn't have anything. She was going through her own depression. She was on drugs and she was an alcoholic, but she loved her big sister. I stayed there up until Christie came; then after a half an hour of being there with her, I left.

I would throw my 2 Pac Makevelli C.D. on and turn to the song, "Crazy."

I'd put it on repeat and walk all the way home listening to it. Once I got through Vailsburg Park, I would see my brother Dawoo and we would walk to get some weed, coke, and a forty. We would get high in the back of my building, before I would go in the house to Sonita. She would know when I came back there because I always listened to 2 Pac. She would just smile at me, speak to my brother, then finish what she was doing. Dawoo told me right then, "Hakeem, you gonna have to fuck Bernard up for real, at least for your moms." I said, "Oh no doubt. He will get his."

I went upstairs and talked with Sonita. She took me back that night by playing a tape we used to listen to when we were in V.A. She always had a way of cheering me up.

The third day was Thursday. I still haven't been to work, due to the fact, I have my mom on my brain.

Sonita goes to work and I told her, "I'll check her tonight."

When I get to the hospital this time, my mother's younger brother is there.

I felt real good to see him.

My moms looked out for him the most, out of her two brothers.

She took me with her to prison to see him and everything; even though she hated going.

But, I used to pester her to take me to see him. I looked up to him.

My Aunt Kim and my cousin Valerie were there.

All of us were talking and passing time with my mother.

Then, Bernard came up and my Uncle Tyrone called me out of the room in order to tell me, "Leave Bernard alone. He's going through so much with my sister dieing."

I flipped and said,

"Fuck Bernard, feelings; what about mines?

What about my mothers! She's fighting for her life and you're concerned with Bernard.

You know what, I could spit right in your face for what you just said to me.

Tyrone, fuck you and Bernard!" Afterwards I started walking down the hall because I knew if I had stood there I would have swung on my uncle. My cousin Valerie asked me where I was going as she was coming out of my mother's room. I just kept walking.

She caught up with me and asked me, "What was going on?"

I told her, "I was hurt now because both of my uncles had turned on my mother, who is their sister. I couldn't believe it!"

Valerie calmed me down and we walked back to my mother's room.

Bernard and Tyrone were talking.

Then, Tyrone said he was leaving, so Valerie said, "I'm going downstairs with you so I can smoke a cigarette.

Bernard started rubbing my moms arm saying, "Yeah, she is so weak; yes, so weak.

I snapped, "No she's not! Why the fuck is you saying that around my moms, what are you trying to do, crush her spirits?"

He said, "Oh, no I can tell." I said, "Tell what?" Then he said,

"Well, your moms wanted me to give you a thousand dollars out of her money.

So I'm giving it to you in front of her. I know you wouldn't do this for me." Then I said, "Man, I don't want no money!"

Bernard then said,

"No, your moms told me to give it to you."

I said, "Whatever." Kim was right there looking, with a smirk on her face. He gave me the thousand dollars.

I said to myself, I'm still going to fuck you up!

After that he left. Then, Kim told me how he gave Tyrone $300.00 to intimidate me.

But it didn't work.

Christie came in and did her shift with our mother. I loved Christie for that. She kept me up when I was feeling down.

I left, put in 2 Pac and did my normal once I got to Dawoo. Then, I went upstairs and talked to Sonita.

My mind was truly fucked up.

I just lost three female cousins the year before, my grand aunt, five friends and three male cousins since this year began, and now my mother is fighting for her life. My girl is holding me down, even though she is going through a tough time being pregnant for the first time. She's two months and she is already looking at her stomach like, it's big right? I busted out with laughter, and said, "Your stomach look the same." (smile) Then she said, "No it don't," with a smirk on her face.

We laughed about it, while we watched a movie. Sonita really had the power to take my pain away, and put my heart and soul at ease. No matter how hard the task, her belief in me, would push me to conquer my demons. Whatever perplexed me.

She had a loving, helpful, concerned, and compassionate way about her.

The fourth day was Friday. By then several family members had been to the hospital to see my moms, since every one knows. Valerie came to pick me up so we could go be with my moms. On our way down to the hospital, Valerie asked me if my Aunt Debby knew? I said, "No, not to my knowledge." Valerie said, "Well I know where she lives, let's go to her house first. Ironically, that's just what we did and she was there stressing some things she and Ed were going through. Aunt Debby was the type who took up for the whole family. She would fight men for her brothers, and girls, for her sisters. Debby was the oldest, toughest, and the tallest.

She was so happy to see us. She said that nobody ever comes to visit her and the main reason is because she lives in Dayton Street Projects, where you will get robbed, beat down, or shot up if you don't know any strong people down there.

We all knew Debby and our side of the family was strong, but if they weren't home when you went through, your ass got a chance of being a victim.

She asked us, why we had come and then the happy faces turned into frowns.

Valerie and I couldn't hold it back any more.

We told Debby everything that was going on.

She went hysterical, started screaming and crying.

She kept saying, "They killed my only son just 5 months ago, now Bernard has done this to my little sister! I want to see her; Valerie, please take me to see my sister!"

I told Debby, "Look, I'm going to take a walk to get some beer. Let's just have a drink or two, I got dough."

She said, "That's fine nephew, but I'm going to walk with you.

Valerie said, "Me too. I said, "I'm good." But Debby insisted.

We got our drink on and reminisce about our family. Then, we got into Valerie car and went to the hospital.

When Debby saw my mother, she was in tears. She kept screaming, "Bernard did this to you, oh he is gonna burn in hell! he's gonna burn in hell!" Kim was there as usual, filling me and Valerie on my mother's progress.

From what she shared with us, my mother was doing better. The doctors thought she would be dead by now, but she is showing her drive to live. By us coming to see her, it was helping her recovery. Then Bernard came in.

Debby said, "Look Bernard, I want all you to leave so I can spend some time with my sister.

So Kim, Valerie and me started going to the door. But Bernard said, "I aint going any where, this is my wife."

Valerie said, "Damn Bernard, Debby is just finding out; give her some time with her sister." I said, "Word, what's wrong with that?" So, Bernard said, "I'm not leaving." then he pushed Valerie aside.

I lost it and couldn't hold it back any longer.

I grabbed Bernard and punched him in the face. He fell immediately. I picked him up and slammed him on the floor. Then, I started punching him in the ribs. He started screaming for his life. Debby started screaming, "Shut your bitch ass up!"

While I was punishing him, he managed to grab the emergency cord and the nurses and doctors ran into the room.

One nurse ran back out and called security. The police came and pulled me off him. Bernard was pleading for his life. "Please don't kill me; don't kill me."

My Aunt Kim scream out, "No, don't take my nephew, Bernard started it!

It wasn't him, it wasn't him!"

Debby was flipping on the cops, too. She was so mad at Bernard that she back smacked him to the ground! And he screamed, "Lock them all up, they jumped me, they jumped me!"

Kim said, "He's lying!" But, they wouldn't listen. The ill part of the whole thing was, this all took place right in front of my mother.

When they started pulling me out the room, I looked back at my moms and she looked at me, and nodded her head yes and she said in a soft voice, "Thank you, son."

The police started grabbing Debby and Valerie.

Kim kept telling them, "We didn't start it. It was Bernard."

He yelled at Kim, "Shut up!" And Debby said, "I know you ain't screaming at my baby sister! I'm going to get you! On my mother's grave, I'm a get you!"

I was just listening, zoning out. I was never built for the arguing. I felt good as hell because I fucked Bernard up. Some tension was off me, but I knew once I got out of this situation I was gonna fuck Bernard up for real and no one will be able to save him.

They took us to a holding cell they had in the hospital. I was shocked!

I didn't know about a jail in the hospital.

There were two holding cells. They put Debby and Valerie in one, and they put me in the other. Debby and Valerie were drunk and mad as hell. They started arguing with each other to the point, they started fighting one another. I yell at them and told them,

"Cut that shit out, Bernard is the enemy, not us! We don't have any reason to be fighting each other." Valerie said, "I know, but that's Debby hitting on me first, and I ain't having that!"

Debby said, "You shouldn't been running your mouth."

I said, "Debby, chill the fuck out alright. My moms is fighting for her life, and we are down here, this shit is fucked up!"

Then Debby said, "You're right Randell, look officer, I want you to give us a report on how my sister is doing every four hours."

The officer said, "I can't promise you nothing, but I'll try."

Then Debby said, "That's all I asked you to do, try mother fucker, try!"

I said, "Debby chill out damn!" Three hours went past with them still arguing, but they weren't fighting any more.

Then, they ended up singing a song from when they grew up. Finally, another officer came in and they let Valerie go.

We were happy about that because we knew we would be next.

I just went to sleep.

Saturday morning the officers switched shifts and the coming on officer didn't know what happened.

He had to give a report to the judge to see if we could be released on our own.

He was telling the judge that all he knew was that a group of people stormed in a husband's wife's room and started beating him up. The husband had to be treated for injuries. So I intervened and said, "Officer, he is my father; it was a family dispute."

So he said, "Oh, Your Honor, I was just informed that the suspect is the husband's son. The fight was over his mother."

The Judge must of have said, "Was the husband still in the hospital?" Because the officer said, "I'm not sure if he is still in the hospital your honor, but can the son and his aunt be released?" The Judge said, "Not until you find out the seriousness of the husband. They will get a bail Monday."

The officer repeated to us what the Judge said and our spirits were crushed.

I just sat down in the corner and stared at the walls. Debby went ahead and explained to the officer what happened.

His heart went out to us because he went to find out about Bernard's injuries.

He was released; they weren't life threatening.

He let us use the phone to call our people.

He even left the cells unlocked. Debby and I had the most deepest conversations in our life.

The officer gave us Jet Magazines to read, plus he checked up on my mother every two hours.

I really grew a new found respect for Newark Cops. Saturday night came and we cracked jokes and talked ourselves to sleep.

Sunday morning I woke up to screaming. Debby kept saying, "Randell get up! Randell get up!" I said, "What happen?" She said, "I asked the new officer, who relieved the white officer, to give me a report on your mother."

I said, "Right and what happen?" Debby said, "The lady called, then she said, "Oh my God, oh my God."

Then she hung up the phone, and walked out. She wouldn't tell me what was said!"

Debby kept crying, saying she wouldn't tell me, she wouldn't tell me, me, me!"

I tried to be calm, but the officer came back with 5 more. I'm trying to figure out, what for. So, I asked, "What's going on?" The female officer said, "You will be informed in a minute, just hang out for a moment right now, though." I knew I was going to see my moms and tell her,

"Where I was slacking as a son, I'm a fulfill as a man."

They told my aunt and me to turn around so that they could cuff us. We complied.

They took us out and we could hear on their walkie talkies, officers asking whether things were okay.

She would call back, it's affirmative. We went to another floor.

The room they sat us in looked like a funeral home. There the doctors informed me right then that my mother has died in peace with no pain. My whole mind went null and void.

I asked the officer, "Can you take me back to my cell now?"

She said, "Yes." The doctor said, "Do you have any questions? I said, "No."

I got up and headed back to the cell.

That night the whole hospital was feeling my pain. My mom had died, and I'm not even on the streets. I couldn't even be by her side!

My last look was when she nodded her head yes and without breath said, "Thank you son!"

It was supposed to be another time, another day; at least for me; just me.

The officers brings a real big dinner. Debby and I appreciated all the cooking they did.

Monday morning the cop from earlier that Saturday came in and checked the static on my moms and when he found out that she died, he was heart broking.

He got on the phone with the judge and he told us he was personally taking us down to the court building.

The judge let us go and gave us a court date to come back. The cop drove us back to the hospital so we could view my mother in the morgue.

However, Perry Funeral Home had already picked her up. Solemnly, we went to the funeral home, but they said my mother wasn't ready to be viewed. I didn't care, I still wanted to see her. I was crying and my heart was broken.

They refused and talked with Debby because they knew her from all the times our family been there.

We left and caught a cab to my house. There, I hugged Sonita and told her what happened.

My Aunt Debby left. I gave her some money so she would be alright.

My brothers found out that I was out and they came to see me, along with my Uncle Naim. They comforted me and later on broke out.

Sonia and I were together looking through my album book. I couldn't hold it no longer, I cried so hard my eyes, jaws and stomach hurt. I had the worse headache in my life.

I went to the funeral on September 5,1997 although, Sonita stayed home and cooked the food.

My cousin Rhonda came over and helped her.

My whole side of the family were there, except for Tyrone and Randy.

They were with Bernard, guarding him from my cousins and me.

We peeped it out and was going to bum rush them, but Valerie told me not to do it. She asked that I let my mother's funeral be in peace. Our family has a history for fighting in this funeral home for the last 15 years.

We eventually chilled out. I read the program they give you and it was all wrong. I had to walk out.

After the funeral, the whole family met back at my house.

I really felt good that they chose to come by and support me

My whole world was upside down. My moms was the cornerstone to my existence.

I never felt more alone in my life. I was traumatized, and began having nightmares.

Any little thing would tick me off and I would want to fight.

I stayed both high and drunk every other day.

I figured, if it wasn't everyday I wasn't a weed head or an alcoholic. That was just my reasoning.

Sonita stood by me through it all.

Now, after losing my mother, I really knew how she felt.

I actually looked up to her and felt sorry for her at the same time, why, because she lost her moms when she was 6.

I was 27 when my moms left and I didn't know how to function.

In October of '97 I finally got in contact with my children's mother. She told me she didn't have any problem with me seeing the children. She said, "They miss you so much." I told her, "I miss them too." I need to see them so I can have someone to love. My role as daddy really took on a new meaning when my moms left. I realized that without me they would have a hard time growing up right. Sonita and I planned a trip down to VA to see my children and her family. We went in November.

We stayed at my cousin Jazz's house. We had fun with him and his family. Then he broke out and went back to Jersey.

He let me hold his red BMW so that I could take Sonita to see her family.

Then, we went to see my children.

They were staying on St. Julian St in Norfolk. When I rode down the block, Sonita spotted Naquasha running down the block.

We blew the horn and she saw us. She and the other children started running back towards the house.

When I got to the house, it was nothing like Susan had told me. It looked abandoned.

I was shocked to the point that I couldn't believe this was the house!

I told my daughter to go get her mother and she did.

When her moms came to the door, she looked terrible. Then, Rahshon and Randell came to the door.

They needed haircuts and Naquasha needed her hair done. Susan wanted me to come inside, but I told her "I'll stay out side." She insisted. She showed me their rooms and it was awful. It looked like a trash dump. I couldn't understand how she thought she was impressing me by showing me this dump. I couldn't take it, so I went back outside.

Sonita was in the car waiting. Susan said, "That's why you wanted to go outside, for that bitch?"

I said, "Don't even fuck with her, she didn't do shit to you. Just get the kids dress."

She said, "They are." I said, "What!"

Susan said, "You buy them some clothes!"

I said, "Okay Susan, okay." Then I told the kids, "Come on lets go." We left, took them to the store and bought them some clothes. We went to Jazz's house and had a ball. When the weekend was over, we took them back and Susan wasn't there. We stayed there for a hour, and no one showed up.

When I got in contact with her she said, "Take them with you."

I didn't have any money to bring them up. But Jazz Western Union me the money to bring them back.

We had to catch the Greyhound back and we almost missed it. They were happy as hell! They talk Sonita and me to deaf. They had us laughing and crying the whole time.

I knew right then my children were survivors.

We enrolled them into school and they were doing well.

Then three months later, Susan came to my house and said,

"She want them back." I told her no, and further stated,

"When they get out of school for the summer, they can stay with you, but I'm not taking them out of school when they are doing well. You have to wait."

She said, "No, I don't want to wait, I want them to go with me to New York to see my family." I looked at her and said,

"They can see them but not right now. They have school, plus you just don't come into my house and make demands!

We haven't heard from you in three months. Dig, I'm going to let you see them because I would never deprive you of that, but they ain't leaving with you."

She was mad as hell. She wanted to show out. She threatened to call my probation officer and tell him about when I went to V.A. to get the kids; knowing I can't leave the state. I bluffed her out and told her I don't give a fuck.

However I really did. I compromised with her because I didn't want any drama.

Sonita was having my baby and I planned on being there.

I told her, "They can go with you to see your family and I'll be there Sunday to pick them up." She said, "Bet."

She chilled at my house with them and we eventually asked them if they wanted to see their family, and they said, "Yeah."

Rahshon said, "We can come back home?" I said, "Of course."

I said to myself, this boy is smart as hell, he wants to make sure he gets his answer in front of daddy.

They went that night and spent all of Saturday there. Sunday came and I went to get them that night.

Sean, Naquasha, and Randell Jr. wanted to stay, however Rahshon wanted to go and rolled with me.

They switched them out of school; now they are Brooklyn residents.

When I brought only Rashon back, Sonita asked me, what happen and I told her.

It actually took a load off of her.

She was their mother when they were there, and all my kids respected and loved her.

It was Rhashon and us. That's when I told him that Sonita is having a baby, and that he was going to have a little brother. He was happy. He started hitting us with, "Where do babies come from?"

Now mind you, this young fella is only 4 years old. Sonita and I laughed about it and just told him the truth.

He was amazed. He said, "So I can be the first one to tell Randell Jr?"

"Word, son, word." was my reply.

Sonita and me started planning our move back to V.A. She hated it in New Jersey because people seemed to die so quickly.

It bothered her if I would leave out because she didn't know if I would make it back.

Subsequently, I understood her fears.

She didn't want to raise her child in that atmosphere. I went with her to her doctor's appointments and stayed in the house more with her. As the later months came, she would cry a lot for no apparent reason.

Her past used to haunt her because she did not have a mother or father.

I did my best to assure her that it wasn't her fault. I told her, "Stop blaming yourself for your father not doing his job. You are a wonderful person, and things will get better for you; plus, you will get to see your mother in the new system. Jehovah will wipe away all of your tears and death will be no more." I turned to the scripture at Revelation 21:3,4

She read it and felt better knowing Jehovah will make a way. As the months went by, she was able to feel the baby kick inside her stomach. She would smile from ear to ear. She always had that kind of smile that would light up a room.

We went to the doctor for the ultrasound and I could see that our son looked just like her.

This was the happiest time of our life.

We brought New Year's in together and the months started flying.

In February and March we had two false alarms.

I told her, "Girl you will know it's the real deal. Then, on March 24,1998, her water broke around 5:00 o'clock. The water, as well as a sharp pain woke her up.

She tried to wake me, although I was not having it.

I told her, "It's probably a false alarm." I was drunk from the night before.

My head was hurting and all I wanted to do was sleep.

She said, "I don't think so baby." Then, she took a shower, got dressed and started walking around the house.

I was asleep the whole time. She tried to wake me. although I couldn't budge.

Consequently at 6:30 in the morning, she walked around the corner to my grandma's house and asked her for help.

They came back to the house and got me up at 6:54 in the morning I got Rahshon up and we bounced.

My grandma cursed me out the whole way there. She was saying,

"Boy, if the girl told you a hundred times her water bust, you get your ass up!"

I kept saying that, "I was sorry, and it's my fault, Sonita. I'm up now, I'm up!"

We arrived a little pass 8 am, at Beth Israel Hospital, in Newark New Jersey.

We went in and got her a walking chair.

I started pushing her to the delivery floor, as we rolled down the hall grandma said,

"I'm taking Rahshon with me so he can eat. You take care of that girl, alright. I said, "Yes ma."

I went into the room with her. She was scared and in pain. I held her hand and she squeezed the hell out of mine.

They drugged her up and she started to feel better.

Then after an hour the pain started to kick in again. I told them to give her some more. They said, "In a minute."

I was rubbing her back and trying to comfort her.

I could tell it really helped.

All of a sudden, she grabbed me and said, "I'm hurting baby, do something!"

I shouted to the nurse, "Give her the stuff now!"

She said in a calm voice; "o.k. this will put her to sleep."

I didn't care. It worked and she was out.

Afterwards I called all my people and told them that my girl was about to have my seed!

I left and went down to Bergen St to see who was out. Afterwards, I hit the park and then headed back to the hospital. By then she was just waking up.

The doctors told me that she was 7 centimeters so they took us in another room.

They had to cut her a little and on the second push, Jehdiah was here. He didn't say a word.

No crying or anything. You can see he is alive because he was blinking, but no crying. I said to myself I got the coolest son. He looks just like his mother beautiful as ever.

They were trying to take him in before she could see him and she flipped. Looking tired and weak, she said,

"Hold up, let me see him. Baby, do he have all his fingers and toes?"

I chuckled inside because I remembered we were watching a television show that documented nurses stealing babies. Therefore, Sonita wanted to make sure she saw her child.

I was feeling her. I went with them to band and clean him.

Jehdiah was here, my first born son by her has arrived!

She called her sister Kim and told her.

Afterwards, I talked to Kim for a minute. Sonita went to sleep.

My grandma came back and I went home and clean up. Rahshon helped me.

He kept saying, "I can't wait to see my brother."

We even decorated the room for Jehdiah.

I went back the next day and she was breast feeding him. She looked so happy; even though she was worn out.

The following day, they were coming home.

Everybody came through to see him and Sonita made sure people wash their hands before touching him. Our child was shining.

SEVEN
The Departure.

JEHDIAH WAS A GOOD baby and Sonita looked out for him from the door.

She would get up in the middle of the night and just stare at him.

We took him to his appointments together and Rahshon was a big help.

He loved his little brother.

We let Rahshon feed Jehdiah and everything.

Whenever we needed a break, Rahshon was there.

Then, in May of 98, Susan comes to my house.

She wanted to take Rahshon to Brooklyn with her, but Rahshon didn't want to go instead he wanted to stay with us. Susan was heated because I didn't let her into my house and besides Rahshon didn't want to see her. Steamed as ever, she left. Three days later, the police were banging at my door, hard as hell. I heard one of them say, "Lets kick the door in." Sonita is scared to death and I'm mad as hell! Nonetheless I opened the door and screamed." What the fuck are ya'll banging on my door for?" They said, "Is Rahshon Barkley here?"

I said, "Yes he's my son? Why?"

They came in and said they had to see him it was an emergency. I asked, "Emergency? Its 7:00 in the morning!" "There's nothing wrong with my son!" They came in and I took them to the back room where Rahshon was sound asleep.

They called in to the dispatcher and reported that, the boy is fine. It's a false alarm.

I said, "Who called you and said something is wrong with my child?"

They said, "We don't have all that information yet;

All we know is the call came in from Brooklyn N.Y.P.D.

That the child's life is in danger."

They woke him up and asked him whether he alright? He said, "Yes."

The police smiled and said, "You can go back to sleep."

As for you Mr.Randell Barkley, its a warrant out for your arrest.

You have to go with us."

Sonita said, "What did he do? "

They said, "It's nothing major, he'll probably get a bail; its for traffic court."

I said, "I can't believe this shit! Susan did this shit I know it!"

Sonita and Rahshon started crying. They let me get dressed and we left.

Sonita told my grandma what happened.

I'm locked up for some traffic shit. I thought to myself, it's got to be from 92 sometime because I've been gone since '94.

Now I'm back sitting in Irvington Jail. I'm broke, so I know I can't make bail.

Sonita is now going to try to borrow money from my family.

I know they ain't going to help.

Three hours passed and the police called my name. I answered. They took me out the cell and, to the Sergeant's office.

He asked me, "Do you know a woman named Susan?" I said, "Unfortunately, she's my wife. He said, "Oh."

"Does she know where you live?" I said, "Yes, she's been to my house several times, as a matter of fact there's a restraining order out on her now, is she here?"

He said, "Don't worry about that right now. Is your son by her home?"

I said, "Yes, he's with my girlfriend." He said, "Thank you for your honesty Mr. Barkley.

Your wife is here and she claims she just found out where you live and you refused to let her see her son?"

I said, "That's bullshit, she was just at my house three days ago!

I refused to let her take my son to Brooklyn because he is scared of her and he didn't want to go."

He said, "You have a restraining order out on her though? I said, "Yes." He then said, "Stay right here." He left and came back. He said, "Do you know where it is?"

I said, "Yes."

He told me to call my house and have my girlfriend give it to one of my officers.

I did that. They held Susan in the precinct until the officer returned.

They served her with the restraining order and told her that if they catch her in Irvington they were going to lock her up; plus she couldn't get her son back because he's in the custody of his father, now split.

The sergeant told me he knew something wasn't right with her story, and they felt bad after Brooklyn police called them to respond to a false alarm.

They put me back in my cell and I went to sleep. The next morning I got a bail.

It was really a fine I owed the courts.$750.00

Around 8 O'clock that night they call me again. They said that I post bail. I couldn't believe it. I knew I didn't have any money.

When I walked out, there was Sonita waiting for me with her beautiful smile. I said, "Where did you get the money?"

She said, "I asked everybody in your family and no one would help except your grandma; she gave me some money, but it wasn't enough. Miraculously this morning your income tax return came back for $1,000.00

I went back to grandma and asked her, could your uncle Lowl give me the money and he could hold your check until you get out. He gave me the money."

Sonita told me she walked up here, because that's all she had.

Right then, I said, "You know what, I'm a marry you."

Sonita said, "Whatever, you've been saying that for three years now.(smile)

I said, "Well this time I'm a make you a believer."

We walked to my grandma's house to pick up Rahshon and Jehdiah.

Then we went home and made love.

The next day I cashed my check to pay grandma and Uncle Lowl back.

I gave them my thanks for looking out for me.

Two weeks later, I went to pick Rahshon up from school.

They told me his mother had picked him up. I was furious! I said to myself, this girl just doesn't stop.

I go to the courts with what happen they tell me they can't do anything until Rahshon is in their jurisdiction.

This bullshit here was giving me a headache. I left V.A. to get away from their mom. Then, she comes up here to start shit.

Sonita and I was fed up by now. She said, Well, Susan is up here somewhere.

Let's move back to V.A, I don't want to raise our child up here anyway.

We planned our move then, but there was still some unfinished business that I had to take care of first.

My brothers wanted me to do things with them, but I limited my time with them.

Sonita and I grew closer and closer together. Meanwhile a lot of my friends started dieing really fast.

It shocked her, and she told me she wanted to raise Jehdiah down South.

In June of '98 I put her on the bus with Jehdiah and they went back down South to stay with her grandfather.

I promised her, I'll be moving back in two months.

My goal was to hit the block hard for two months and reunite with her. I put the move in motion and started getting dough. I was really stressed out though, my mom died 10 months ago and now the love of my life is back in V.A.

I stayed high and drunk. My apartment became the spot.

All my family came over and we were constantly partying and wilding out.

I would write Sonita to keep her informed.

She told me she hated living with her grandfather because her aunt and uncles kept the house dirty.

She didn't want Jehdiah to crawl on the floor because it stayed filthy.

I told her to just be patient, and I'll be down there soon.

Sonita would call me at my grandma's house and we would talk for hours.

She told me she missed me very much and she needed me down there.

I told her, "I'll be down there two visit you and my son in August.

Then she said, "It's something else?" I said, "What?" She said softly,

"I'm pregnant again." I thought to myself damn, Jehdiah aint one yet. I got to step up my game.

I caught the bus down there and my cousin Jazz picked me up. I filled his car up with gas and we went out to breakfast. He saw the knot of money I had and was amazed. He said, "I see your getting it, your getting it!!"

"I said, "A little something, something."

We laughed and carried on. I dropped my bags at his house and got in contact with Gwen, my step brother's moms.

I had her take me to Sonita's house. She was three months pregnant. We all had fun.

It was Sonita, her grandfather,Gwean, her uncle Robert and me. We talked and laughed, plus we took pictures.

Jehdiah looked just like Rahshon when I saw him.

I stayed down there at her grandfather house. I slept right on the couch.

I really wanted to take her to a hotel, but we couldn't get know one to take us.

We would've wasted unnecessary money on cabs and buses if we tried to get there on our own.

I preferred for my son and girl to get that money.

When it was time for me to go, Sonita would always cry. She would always say,

"I love you bay".

That was her nickname for me. Out side of being her Boo.

I felt her realness each time. The lump would be in my throat because I wanted to cry too.

However, I smiled, hugged, and kissed her, then I bounced.

When I get back to the Bricks, the beast in me comes out.

The hate, the pain, the struggle, and anger are written all over my face the same as everyone else.

I'm still in my apartment and doing my thing. I met this girl through one of my cousins and we ended up sleeping around. That was bothering me because, I broke our bond, and Sonita was still being faithful to me.

Even though she didn't know. I started getting higher and higher; just messing up money.

When I called, Sonita would scream on me.

After a while, she knew something was wrong.

All the money I was supposed to send was being cut in half.

She told me to bring my ass or she is going to move in with her sister.

I said to myself, "What the hell am I doing, this is my girl with my child and we are about to have another one."

I cut the girl I met off, and got back on my plan to move.

September rolls around and I'm on the block hard.

As soon as I made $2,000.00 I went down South.

I got us a hotel room for a week. I got in contact with my cousin Vernon.

He already has a company down here; plus he promise me work, that way I could take care of my family.

All I needed to do was find us an apartment. The second day I went to work with him.

On the fifth day we found an apartment on 14th Bay in ocean view. Judy Boone was renting it out. So we went to her office on Chesapeake Blvd in Norfolk VA, and told her, "I just moved down here, and we are living in a hotel.

I got a job and I just need a spot for my family."

It work out. I get a call from my grandma. She tells me my son Sean called and told her where they were.

I felt good about everything falling in place.

I told Sonita, "I had to go back up top this one time so that I could locate my other children." She was hurt and stressed out.

The doctors had said that she was carrying this baby very low, and her placenta wasn't strong enough to hold the baby.

As a result she had to take it easy. We got the keys to our place, but Sonita refused to move in without me.

She stayed with her grandfather once I left to return to New Jersey.

I go to the place my children were and Susan's sister welcomes me in with open arms.

She tells me how Susan is still getting high, plus she is still with Poo.

Poo is suppose to be dragging her down. I really didn't care, because I was going on with my life. I just wanted my children. Tasha made very sure it was clear that they could go with me whenever, because Susan wasn't coming to see them.

Why should she deprive me?

I was happy with that information, so I went back to New Jersey and partied with my brothers.

I ended up at some girl's house with my brother. I didn't know where I was.

She cooked us breakfast and we left. I asked him, "Did we gangbang her or what?"

He said, "No Hakeem, this one was all me, your drunk ass went to sleep.(smile)

When we arrived at grandma's house she was mad at me. I asked her, "What did I do?" She said, "Sonita grandfather was calling here all night for you. Sonita is in the hospital; she lost the baby!"

My mind went blank. If only I would've stayed down there, it probably wouldn't have happened. I felt terrible and stupid.

Here I am partying because I found my other children and my girl lost our baby.

I was in another world; This one was very foggy and strange.

Josiah was born October 2,1998, and died the same day.

I wasn't even there.

I called to the hospital. Sonita just cried on the phone, blaming herself for losing the baby. She was more afraid and stressed out about me being mad at her, than the fact that I wasn't there.

She told me her family was trying to console her by saying,

"Josiah died for a reason ,God wanted him back."

That made her angry instead because she couldn't believe God would do something like that.

She called Sister Young, who is a Jehovah's Witness and she helped her see that these things originate from Adam and Eve sinning against Jehovah God. Thus, bringing sin and death into the world.

However, Mrs. Young reassured her that she will see her son Josiah in paradise on earth in the near future.

I was too out of it for God's reason or justification. My question, is why mine?

It's my fault and I needed to get back down there. So, I did.

I moved us into our apartment and I started working with Vernon again.

Sonita was very depressed about losing our baby.

She would cry in the middle of the night.

I was tired as hell, but I'd be up with her.

I felt that she is so strong to go through all of this, plus she is young.

I don't know of any girls her age dealing with the things she dealt with.

My mother was dead and I still didn't know whether I was coming or going.

November came around and it was my daughter's birthday. Tasha had already asked me to bring a cake or something because Susan wasn't anywhere to be found.

I told Sonita I was going up for that and I'll be back in one week

Like usual, she didn't want me to go.

However, I was going. I went to New Jersey first to buy Naquasha a cake and some balloons.

It was November 6,1998, when I took her gift's to Brooklyn and we celebrated!!!!

Their mom wasn't there. It was just the rest of the family.

When I saw Sean, he had a busted lip, he told me he was jumped by some kids. Looking at his face made me feel bad for him. I didn't want my children dealing with that.

Nonetheless, it was their reality. I told him, "Tuesday when you go to school, I'm going with you and he was shocked.

I told Sonita I was going to be up here for one extra week. She wasn't hearing it.

However I stood by my decision. My son Sean didn't have anybody. I wanted him to know he had people.

I went back that Tuesday and the kids were there, but Tasha wasn't.

Sean said, "Once she come back, we can go?"

I said, "Word."

It was a knock at the door. They didn't know who it was.

I answered it and it was a lady from social services.

She came by to inspect the house because Tasha is about to be granted with custody of my children.

I said, "Hell no she ain't!"

I told the lady that I was their father. Her records indicated that I was either deceased or incarcerated for life.

I told the lady, "I'm right here. Ask those kids who their daddy is?"

They told her. In the meantime Tasha comes home. I had been there for at least two hours when this lady comes, and she stayed for about one hour.

Now Tasha is raising hell; acting like she hated me or something. I had to speak the truth.

I told her that I was just down here last week, and you weren't acting like this.

She kept telling me to get out. I wouldn't leave until the social worker made sure I was in the report.

She told me to go to the Brooklyn Court House and tell them you contest the decision because you are their father.

I did that and dreaded telling Sonita I had to stay a extra week. I know she is going to be mad. Eventually I told her and she was pissed. However, I had to stay and fight for my children.

They shouldn't have to go through this, but they mother started it.

I definitely planned on finishing it.

I went to court on the 12th of November.

They gave us another court date for December 15,1998.

Tasha was mad as hell because they granted me visitation.

I contacted Sonita and told her what happened. I said, "I'll be on the bus tonight."

I came home and Jehdiah bum rushed me once I walked in.

She gave me a hug and kiss after Jehdiah got his time.

We talked the day away. She informed me on Jehdiah singing skills, and how smart he was. Sonita would have me weak with laughter, when she talk about the guys around the house who always sweat her. I loved and respected her loyalty and honesty.

That night I rented some Blockbuster movies and we all cuddled up and watched movies.

I continued to work with Vernon, while Sonita held down the house and took care of Jehdiah.

In our spare time, we would play Casino and two hand Spades. We took a lot of pictures of Jehdiah, and played music. We also took walks at the beach when it was nice.

We were so happy together. Time went fast and my visitation started the first weekend in December. Therefore I had to leave.

Sonita tried to hold a smile, but I could tell she hated me leaving.

I left on the last Greyhound and arrived at Newark Penn Station in the morning.

I linked with Dawoo and David Glover.

We did the usual thing, then I went to New York to pick up my children.

My visitation was from 12pm to 5pm.

It took me 2 hours to get the kids to New Jersey, on the way they had so much to talk about.

I took them to the movies and before you knew it, it was time to take them back.

No one wanted to go back and I was trying my hardest to explain to them that I don't want to take ya'll back, however the courts made this temporary arrangement so it wouldn't be a problem when I get full custody again.

They didn't understand, all they knew was they were with me now and they didn't want to go back.

I asked my grandma what to do? She said, "Call Tasha and ask her if it's alright if they stay for the whole weekend."

I called Tasha and asked her, she said, "It was cool."

So they stayed. They were happy as hell.

I felt bad that I had to ask her sister about my own kids.

The next day, all their cousins came over and they had a blast!

Then, I took them back. They hated that part.

When I got there, Tasha wasn't there.

I waited 1 hour for her to get back, although she never showed. I'm thinking, does she leave the kids like this all the time?

I knew I had to get back because the courts were under the pretense that I lived in New Jersey; however I lived in V.A. and I had to work Monday at a new job I had just gotten.

I told the kids, "I got to go, ya'll behave and I'll call you later."

But Rahshon wasn't having it, he was on my pants leg.

He said, "I don't want to stay and he started crying."

I couldn't take it no more. I told myself forget it, he's rolling.

He's only 4 years old. He can't understand.

To make him know, that no one could keep him from me, I took him and told my other children to chill.

They were sad and they ask me, "You're going to come back right?" I said, "Yes."

I left and went back to my grandma's house.

I explained to her what happened. She suggested that I call Tasha to let her know.

I wasn't going to tell her shit but I called. She was there.

I asked her, "Do you have a problem with Rahshon staying with me?" She said, "No, I know he miss and love you, its cool."

I said, "I'll keep him until our next court date; that would be in two weeks."

She was fine with it. I left that night and took Rahshon with me to V.A.

He was hyped as hell.

We got there in the morning and Sonita was shocked to see him.

Jehdiah knew who he was from the door.

They started playing and I explained to Sonita what happened.

We all had fun. Rahshon was so happy. He said, "This is a nice place, Dad."

I showed him the rooms and it was on.

Meanwhile, I'm working two jobs and Rahshon is helping Sonita out with Jehdiah.

Sonita took Rahshon and Jehdiah to her grandfather's house for a visit.

When Sonita's grandfather saw Jehdiah he was so happy. Jehdiah was his only great grand child who wasn't scared of him. He would play with Jehdiah and feed him all the time. That gave Sonita time to rest, kick back and watch television however, Rahshon didn't know Sonita's grand father so he would follow Jehdiah and Sonita's grandfather wherever he would take Jehdiah. All three of them were having fun.

Then, when Sonita's grandfather started watching television he picked Jehdiah up the best way he could and brought him in the living room where Sonita was.

He told Sonita, "Jehdiah didn't want to be back there."

She just burst out laughing! She realized Rahshon was making sure his little brother was in their eye sight.

All Jehdiah did, once he was comfortable on the floor, was crawl back into his great grandfather's room and Rahshon just followed. Sonita really enjoyed herself that day.

A week later I get a call from my brother Ibn telling me the police kicked in the door looking for Rahshon and me.

He was scared to death because he was hustling then and his works were in the house.

He told me to bring Rahshon back or get in contact with Tasha and see whats the fuck is going on.

He didn't want them coming back and I was steamed.

I called Tasha and she said, "I had to protect myself. If something happened to Rahshon it would be on me."

I said, "That's bullshit, I told you he was going to be with me; you think you're slick.

You told me you didn't have a problem with it."

She said, "Now I do, so bring him back."

I was so mad I wanted to kick Tasha and Susan butt.Tasha said, "When are you going to bring him?" I said, "Saturday."

She said, "What time?" I said, "Around three O'clock."

I went home and told Sonita what happened. She felt bad because she'd been raising Rahshon since he was 5 months old. She knew he would be hurt and she didn't want him to feel like he had done something wrong and that's the reason he's leaving. I understood what she was saying. She was his stepmother and he loved her.

It was on a Wednesday when this happened, so I only had two days left to be with Rahshon.

I figured I'll take him back early, that way she couldn't get me locked up.

I told Rahshon that I had to take him back, but I will be returning to get him.

He started crying! He said, "Why, was I bad? I'm sorry Sonita if I've been bad, but I want to stay with ya'll!"

She said, "No, no, Rahshon; you have been so good baby. You've done nothing wrong.

It's just the procedure we have to do in order to get you, Love Jr. and Naquasha back." He was too hurt to understand.

All he knew was he had to go back to Tasha, whom he hated.

We left that Friday night. He stayed up for the entire six hours; giving me every reason why he should stay with us.

They all were good, smart, and well thought out reasons.

Even people on the bus began asking me why was I taking him back.

I had to explain to strangers why he had to go back and they understood; but how do you get a four- year old to understand the messed up unjust court system that hangs, suspended in the balance of us being together. We got to Tasha's house at 7am

She opened the door half sleep and shocked, because I told her three oclock in the afternoon. But here we are.

I hugged Rahshon and told him to go ahead.

He was both hurt and upset. He didn't even speak to Tasha, he just walked right past her and whispered, "Bye daddy" in a soft tone.

I left with my spirits crushed. I felt like I let my baby son down.

I went to court that Monday and put in another petition for longer visitation.

The judge asked me, "Where was my wife?"

I said, "I didn't know." Tasha wasn't in court so they gave us another court date for January 12, 1999.

The judge said, "Both of them better be in court or he was throwing out the whole case."

I felt good about that. I caught the bus back to V.A. I told Sonita what had happened.

She suggested that, I go to the V.A. Courts and see if they could assist me with this matter. I went on December 22, 1998 and I found out everything Susan did to get custody after I left with the kids and moved to New Jersey with Sonita.

She went to the courts and told them I was locked up in Newark, New Jersey and the children were with her. As a result, she wanted full custody. The case was awarded to her after they attempt to contact me at a bogus Jail she had made up.

They granted her custody! Even though the children were with me the whole time.

The National Certified Counselor assisted me with the investigation and sealed an envelope which included the truth.

That way, once I go to court, I should have no problem getting my children back.

I stayed and worked in V.A. until my court case came up in January.

I was very stressed out myself, at this time because, my life was so messed up.

I'm trying to support my family down South, yet I'm fighting in another state for my other children.

We were barely paying our bills when the lights were cut off on us.

Sonita found out there were mice in the apartment; I had to deal with that also.

She also felt as though I loved my other children more than Jehdiah and she.

Really, I was just confused, hurt, underpaid and overworked.

She didn't want me to go up for the court case either.

I felt like I had come too far to give up now.

The time we spent apart was hard on us.

I arrived in Newark, New Jersey on January 11,1999. I went past Hakeem house so I could find out what's been going on since I left.

He filled me in on our getting high clique.

Later David Glover came through with some goods.

We did the usual and worked on some music.

Hakeem gave me a suit to wear for court and Ibn let me where his diamond ring.

I definitely was looking the part.

I went to court the next day and it was crowded.

I managed to spot Tasha from a distance. She was with two dudes.

They saw me and didn't speak. I was cool with that because I knew, after I showed the judge this letter, they will have a lot to say.

After about two hours of waiting around, they called my name.

As I got up to walk in they shut the door after me and two officers approached me and asked me my name.

I told them and they said I was under arrest for bringing my children to Tasha's house too late. I couldn't believe it!

I said, "Look I have a sealed envelope for the judge from the courts of Virginia.

Just let me give this to him, and take me wherever after the fact."

They said, "We can give it to him for you, but he has already set another court date. Your case wont be heard today, your wife and her sister are here and they've been informed as well." I said, "My wife? I didn't see her with Tasha."

I gave them the letter and they took me into a cell.

The female officer complimented me on my curls and next my suit.

I was digging her style as well, but my mind was stuck on this bullshit I was going through.

The female officer spoke,

"How does a man like you get hooked up with a woman like your wife?

In a jovial manner, she said,

"You can't tell me, she looked better when she was younger!" They laughed.

I said, "I didn't see her out there, so I don't know how she looks now, but she had a nice ass and that's all it took." smile.

From there, they took me out of the building. As soon as we walked out, I saw Tasha and the two dudes.

Then, when I looked harder one of the dudes was actually Susan!

She was skinny as hell with a low cut. I was shocked.

They took me to jail. They looked out for me though, I was fed food from Subway.

I was in my own cell until some Bloods came in.

The female officer didn't want them in the cell with me, but I told her, "I'm alright, you can put them in here."

The white officer wanted to, but she wasn't having it. However there were a lot of them, so three had to come in my cell.

They asked me, "Are you a Lawyer?" I said,

"I'm an inmate like you!" Then they asked me, "What you in for?

I said, "For bringing my kids to their aunt house late of a visit. They were suppose to be back by five, I got them there later than that, so she called the cops, made a report, and they lock me up in court, for violating the visitation order."

One guy said, "Damn, I wish my pops would come see me."

Then, they told me about why they were in there.

They were cool as hell and they looked out for me.

I called my grandma and told her not to tell Sonita about me being locked up.

I knew she was already stressing because I was gone, and I didn't want to add any more.

Three days later I was out.

I had to go back to the court building and file an appeal for longer visitation hours; that way she can't get me like that again. I was asking for the whole weekend.

It was granted two weeks later. I had talked to Sonita about two times since then.

I didn't want to explain what I have to do; I wanted to call when it was done and I'm coming home.

In the meantime back in V.A, she was alone waiting for me, so she began writing back in her Diary.

Heart Broken Soulmate | 95

11:00 pm.
Wednesday - January
1-20-99.

Today, I went to sign a paper stating I never recieved my Last Check from Farm Fresh, Located Behind Pack-a-Sack in Southern Shopping Center. Then I went to Social Services to transfer my case to Norfolk. All Day I've been thinking about Lehdish & My Baby, & My Future. I want to better my life. I know I definetly need all the help from Jehovah God. I want to make all my meetings and become totally spiritually focused. He understands how I feel. My cousin Renee was very helpful in taking me everywhere I had to go today. I finally got a ride home from my Grandfather's House. I've been stranded there since Thursday 14th. That's a very long time in a shitty House. I know all things happen for a reason. My sister Janel showed herself to be all talk as usual. I told my sister Kim what happen. She was upset. This is the thing. It all started when I kept calling MaMa to see if she heard anything about Randell where abouts. She talked to me as though she had grudge against me. I just know the vibe I recieved through the phone wasn't Right. Everyone at my grandfather house told me Randell didn't call. I felt like Either He didn't want to talk to me or He's in trouble.

Page 1   January 28, 1999

Today was a very beautiful day. I almost went to the beach. But I would rather be accompanied by someone on the sand. Randell is in New Jersey now. He didn't even bother to call me back after he hung up on me. Nor the day after, but that's okay. I feel lonely. Back in the day we use to have fun. Well, I always enjoyed Randell's company. I use to check him on the job. And whenever he had jazz on, he would take me somewhere. I know I changed. Maybe he's tired of me and just not telling me, to hurt my feelings. I miss the friendship we use to have. Everything changed when we went to Jersey. Maybe I shouldn't have left & went to pursued school. But I loved him to the point, I couldn't stand seeing him leave. I risked everything just to stay with him. I was scared. And I didn't like the scenery of New Jersey. Or the people. It's dirty, scary, crowded, & dangerous. Being in the house before dark turn me into a couch potatoe. I liked this kid named Cash. She reminded me a little bit of my sister Lisa & my cousin Me-Me. Put together. She always offered to show me all around Jersey & New York & Randell never let me go. Stating she could be crazy or kidnap me. But she was just trying to be a friend to me. She seemed just like family. I felt comfortable talking to her. When I met Fatima she was funny. We use to joke all the time on the clock. But after hours I didn't know she was a freak.

Page 2

So eventually I stopped talking to her. Fatima acted a little like me. Well my Attitude. But I changed. She was still into hanging out all the time smoking weed, drinking, guy friends, just having fun. But somehow I turn into a Good Girl. Still going to the Kingdom Hall. Having my Study with Mrs Johnson. Then being too tired to do anything after work. And after work I was still on the clock having Bhashan & Love to take care of. Cause Love would be with his Brothers with Smithers. I started being a boring person. Talking Plan otherwise & Person Styles were different from everyone & they couldn't SAY things more up that well Like that sort Place. I definitly Did not Fit in. It was hard for me. I wasn't use to the new environment. The new attitude everyone presented. Calling Me Country all the time Got on my Nerves. I wanted to leave after that 2nd Month But didn't say anything. I've been on my porch for about 2 hrs off & on. My thoughts are just wondering around "But I'm just trying to figure out where I went wrong." Why do I still feel Stressed Out & Left Out. I'm on a strick Bed Rest. I can't move too much because the doctor said I'll loose the baby. I want a friend. Someone to take me out & Jehdiah Like Family Outtings. It don't have to be a Sex Thing. Just Talk, Eat, and enjoy each Others Company.

Page 3

I need that!!! My feelings were hurt when my sister changed her mind with a Lame Excuse. She told my sister Kim, Uncle Stanley, Misi, and a couple others that she wanted me to stay with her. She could help me with school, giving me a ride to doctor appointments, help out with child care. And when she said she'll get back with me & Did. I told her I'll accept her offer. She said; she'll pick me up the following weekend. For me to cancel my lease, get the deposit, pack because she was going to borrow this van from someone, make sure I turn off the electricity, & water. So just have everything done by Saturday when she come. When she told me this SUNDAY. I thought to myself, I couldn't believe I was finally moving far away. That I can actually get the ball rolling and have this nice job she was telling me about. Monday I didn't have a ride to get anything done. Tuesday Dwight gave me Bus Fare to take care of everything. So, I felt this strange feeling when I was getting ready to leave. I thought to myself, I said let me call Janel. Just to say Hi & let her know today is the day I can finally get things done. She didn't bother to tell me she really didn't want me & Jendiah to stay. It was this image she was trying to portray that she got it going on and can provide all this help. Because to her I seem, Low Budget.

60 | Page 1

Her excuse was, the night classes were already filled. The G.E.D. classes only had time for Daytime Students, and she wouldn't have a babysitter for me. She wanted us to switch shifts so her or me would be with Jehdiah. She just had an excuse for everything on why I couldn't Go. And she knew all of this when she told me to Pack. That added to my stress. That's why I want to Have someone in my life to make me feel Alive Again. I was in the Worst Position Ever living at Pop House on Chesapeake Blvd But I felt good & had fun. Alecia & Pop Really Did feel like Family. I really liked that White Girl. And it Hurt when the Ugly Nigga told her I said he should be with a sister. Not some White Girl. All these crazy lies. It started because he would tell her go to 7/11 Get some Beer & Blunts, Because she was over 21. And when she leave, he would tell me I'm pretty. That he don't really like that White B. He just like her sucking his Dick. So I told her. And when she questioned him, he flipped the Strip & said I tried to get with him. She Believe him like a Dummy. Then I ended up cutting his sister & cousin up When they tried to jump me For her. Because at the time Alecia's Wrist was Broke

I Will Serve (Jehovah God &)   January 29, 1999
Only Salvation!!! (Jesus Christ)   Thursday.
                                    After Hours (Late)
What Must Be Done. - Sonita's Thoughts

Right now, I'm tired. Physically and Emotionally. I just read the Watch Tower about How do Lead Your Conscience. But the way I feel about how Jehdiah & my Life should & could be better. He's always been in my Life (Since Birth) He's never been apart except if I let him stay the night over my aunt or grandfather's house. But more than a night away, I always kept my baby. He's my only Son, (Baby), & Child. We have a beautiful Bond that's Unseperatable. I don't even want to be threaten that my son will be taken away. Which is why I have to File for Full Physical Custody. I have Earned that right. I'm the only one taking care of my son with help only from My Relatives. I'm going to have another Baby. After this baby I'm getting myself Fixed. I'm taking care of Jehdiah Alone & Now another Baby will be here. (Due Date August 25.) I'm tired of all the B.S. I go through. And I don't like to be Played. My life is being Wasted. But No More!!!!! I'm going to better myself For my Kid's Sake. Starting With School, Pursuing A Career, With A Good Paying Job, and Get A Vehicle. Signed Sonita Brown

Why? - Why Me?

Questions:
1. Why did "My" Mother Have to Die?
2. Why was my Father never in my Life?
3. After we reunited, Why he didn't make the effort to keep in touch.
4. Why didn't I stay in one stable home in my lifetime.
5. Why don't I have any Friends?
6. Why do My Baby Father don't feel the way I Do?
7. Why am I hurting Physically & Emotionally?
8. Why isn't He Dying?
9. Why Does It always drag?
10. Why Don't I have a better lifestyle.

All these questions, Only God can fix. Jehovah God understands, and serving him will cause life to be a very beautiful thing. He promises Eternal Life. Everyday is Happiness.

Grandpa - Julious Dunbar / Grandma - Mildred Amanda Dunbar
Glenda - Mother (Kimberly, Lisa, Eric, Celena, Sonita)
                              Oldest →   Baby Girl
5 Kids   This is an Ideal of the Beginning !!!
4 Girls
1 Boy.   Book is Called (Bounties Of Life), By Sonita Dunbar

63

8 Girls
1) Lucy   Sonita, you better come out the room.
2) Lena   You're going to get your Whipping Sooner or Later. Lisa said.
3) Jack   Sonita screamed loudly, I didn't do it. Eric
4) Alexandra gave me the carrot cake & Kool-Aid Spoon. Meanwhile
5) Doreen   hours went by. Momma picked the locked and pushed
6) Ruth   Sonita away from the Door as she fell asleep.
7) Annette   What a rude awakening. Eric took a Big Spoon
8) Arlene   used for stirring Kool-Aid and dug in the middle
              of the carrot cake Aunt Ruth just brought over for
8 Boys   mama. He gave the cake & spoon to Sonita stating
              it was Okay to eat some, then ran and told mama
David   I Did it by myself. Then I got punished
James   for it. Many good days went by that we were
Kenneth   a Real Family with a tight Bond. Aunt Annette
Stanley   moved in. Those were the funnest times of our
Robert   life. I love her as a Second Mother. My mother
Neal   was in & out of the hospital and I never knew
Wright   why. Then the Day came when she wasn't
Steve   coming out. Annette gathered us together and
              said Aunt Lucy is picking us up later, and
              we will reside with her until my mother get better.
              Changing the only routine we were adjusted too.
              Seeing Mama in the Hospital Every once in
              a while really hurt.

Sunday 31st, 1999 (January)

Jehdiah & I is home relaxing. Right now I'm trying to organize my thoughts on what I can do to stay an independent mother. My family isn't helping me at all. Why? Because they look for me to give up my home and move back into my nasty Grandfather's home. If I loose my apt. I have no choice but to move into a shelter. I don't want that to happen but my life is at risk. Meaning: Being at my grandfather's home causes me to move more - (Get more active instead of resting). Why? Because the house stay disgusting and there's trash all over the floor. Items that my son could put into his mouth and choke. When you clean up, it gradually gets back messed up. Nobody cleans behind themself. And I can't take it. I rather be in a home with no furniture than a house full of Bums & Nasty People. I want to move far away. To me it wouldn't make any difference. Nobody can help me but me. This area is harder for me to get anything done. I want to start new. New Home, Environment, and lifestyle of Living. I have no money, car, or possesions. Just me and my son. And I promised to do any and everything to help him have the best home.

February

Monday 1st 1999

Today I made the effort to ~~find~~ ~~a~~ shelter to enroll into.

How did my day start?

Well I really didn't get much sleep last night. I haven't actually slept well in weeks. I've mapped out what I want to do with ~~my life~~. But I can't seem to find the right way going about doing (accomplishing) anything. I want to get my G.E.D. — Go to College, take classes ~~in~~ the medical field. Get a good paying job. Own my own House & Car. All these things will benefit my kids to have the finer things of life. But the best thing in life my kids & I can have is serving Jehovah. We will be a family that worship Jehovah God & Jesus Christ.

* FEBRUARY *

Tuesday 2nd, 1999

I wish Randell would be honest with me. The silent treatment he gives me hurt alot. He left February 9. The 12th He was suppose to go to court in reference to the kids. But that's every month. You can't go to court for the same thing every month. For 6 months total. He're suppose to go half-n-half on the Rent. He combined our money to move in the Apt. in October. November I paid $265 towards the rent while all he gave was $30. That month he bought a radio, Hair Product, Speaker & Etc. From a Crack Addict. He had an argument, He left and claimed he lost $20. Then he went out with his So called Friends & Blew the rest of his money. Dec. He went to New Jersey claiming to Pick-Up Financial Assistance money & spent it on his kids. I didn't see any of the money. He came back with No Money when it was suppose to be Vice Versa. Working & getting paid every week. Randell only contributed $95 towards the rent. January ($95) Less than Half Rent. Running Back to Jersey. He hasn't returned. He left Jan. 9. Called me 2 times at my grandfather's house. Still running Bullshit Excuses. I'm fed up. My Electric Bill is $413. / Water $63. P.S.E.H. $273 (Phone?) I have to find out $800 / Then worry about Phone Later.

413
63
273
$749

- February -
Wed 3rd 1999

Today I did my hair in Flat Twist. Then I went to the phone to call Annette. I told her my 3 options. To move in with my friend Robin, Ask Uncle David to stay with him, or go to a shelter. She said David stay with someone. Ask Dorrene so I can be close to family. So I asked and she talked me to Death to the Point she aggravated me. The answer was "No" from the door so why keep talking to me about nothing. Then I called Janel. Because yesterday, she told me I better call her so I did. I told her I can stay with Robin for $150. a month. I mention to her about what Dorrene said and that Annette put me up to asking her. So then she asked me do I want to stay with her. I said yeah. Supprizingly. Because she turned me down before. And knew I needed this & that but said nothing. I don't know. But I'll try it Out. (A Sign from God!!!!!)

* February *
Wednesday 3rd, 1999

I know the goals I want to accomplish.
First: Get my Life right with Jehovah God.
Second: Get my Diploma.
Third: Prepare to establish myself for Jehdiah & Baby. Which means getting a vehicle, Saving money $$
I want to pray alot more, not for only things needed, But to form a better relationship with God.
I also need to work on becoming a better person, with patience, and have a sweet personality.

Saturday February 6, 1999

Today is a brand new & beautiful day. Jehovah has allowed another day of life. I pray for his guidence, And strength. I admit I'm selfish, And have my own view points about certain things. I should try to see things from another persons point of view. When I do, I can relate. But my point comes from a different angle. Why? Because everyone's different. And nobody is perfect. You cannot hold something against a person, because they don't always see things your way. You should come together so both persons agree. Compromise. No 1 Person should have to argue, Or hold angry feelings. You should always try to work things out and stop putting each other down. Remember: Nobody's Perfect. And everybody Needs Love.

— Sonita's Morning Thoughts —

- Evening -

(7) Analysing   Saturday February 6, 1999

I feel you should treat people the way you want to be treated. I realize now from Randell's point of view, how he felt. He said we should work together as a team. Honestly, I didn't want pancakes and eggs. I've been in the house all the time, and that's all I eat. He claimed he's tired of eating ~~out~~, and pressured me to cook. I should've acted better than the way I did earlier. I didn't see all the drama he's been going through, nor understood how he felt. I read his court papers, and the whole situation is messed up. I honestly believe some of the things he told me were lies. How can someone recieve so many court dates, and be locked up for something petty? It doesn't seem right. And here I'm acting stubborn. I'm really sorry. I put myself in his shoes to see how he felt.
So I'm going to adjust and make some changes. That way, there won't be any friction. We both need to come together to compromise and make the right choices together.

February
Tuesday 16th 1999.

Inside I have alot of expectations. And I know the only person that can keep me in true happiness is Jehovah God. I want to have a happy life for myself and my son Jebidiah. He gives me alot of joy. Jebidiah desires alot of attention. I'm very happy to have him as my son. I Love Jebidiah with all my heart. This is a blessing Jehovah gave to me. I want to serve Jehovah God and Jesus Christ. God promises to never leave or forsake you. He watch you as you sleep and protect you from evil.

(73)

Time: Late Night
About 11:00 pm.
February
Wednesday 17th 1999

Sonita L. Duncan.

Today, I went to Social Services. My worker asked me to bring a letter from a family member, stating Randell is not in my home. So I bring the letter. It's been over a month since I've last had Food Stamps. But I don't need, nor have to put myself through all the drama of trying to recieve Stamps. By me being on bed rest, she wants a letter from someone who visited me at my home. And a letter from Randell stating he comes to see me every once in a while, and if he gives me money, How Much? She's just trying to give me a hard time, So forget it. I'd rather work for mines, and Put Jehdiah in Day Care. I don't need the stress, nor worry about asking anybody else to write a letter for me like I'm a little kid. She checked with Judy Boone, so she know Randell wrote out the money order from February. And she called Dwight asking him alot of questions. I don't need a social worker trying to be a Detective and figure out my Life. I cut all those Strings Loose.
I've called Randell twice today. He didn't page me or anything.
Jesus Loves Me, This I know, For the Bible tells me so. Little One to Him Belong, They are Weak, But He is Strong. Yes, Jesus Loves Me. Repeat 2 More Times. — For the Bible Tells Me So.

- 8:11 AM -

Friday 27th 1999 February

My feelings are heavy on my chest. Actually, I'm fed up with the petty situations I put myself through. I honestly believe it's best for me to live alone. I don't want to be in a relationship, especially when a person can't understand how I feel. I've been patient, time and again. I'm not saying, ~~I~~ ~~...~~ But if you leave out of state for long periods of time, you can at least make the effort to call me once a day. That's the way I see it. I never know what's going on with Randell. Yet, I can't accomplish anything either. I should've moved with my sister. I really feel bad, that I gave the opportunity up. Why did I? Because, my feelings get disturb when Randell's in my presence. He talked me out of leaving. — I just want my own place. I'm tired of living with other people. Or sharing an apartment, especially when I pay more than half. And I'm very tired of being lied too. Why do people have to lie to me? I'm not God or a High Been Person that holds their life in my hand. I can't tell when he tells the truth or not anymore. I'm tired of it. Is it me? I want to honestly know what I do wrong in a relationship. I cook, clean, keep my sex in good health, and I'm respectful. I'm faithful & honest. Why can't I do better? I probably need to do logical research.

(75)

Question?:

In my home I always pay attention to the materialistic items that make the home more comfortable and easy-going to live in (for instance, extra hygiene products, items for kitchen, wash cloths, towels, sheets, & blankets.) And I'm the only one that supply such items, which it comes out of my pocket. I'm tired of being used. I believe moving into this apartment would be a 50/50 basis. But its not. The other party stays stranded in mother state with no job. Hell, I have a reality check. Jebdish & I is very comfortable living alone. It's relaxing, and peaceful. Now, to maintain peace, I must set up our schedule for the week.

Sunday   Monday   Tuesday   Wednesday   Thursday   Friday   Sat.
"Kingdom Hall" Read Watchtower My Pick Awake My Pick Insight Insight & Wat.
Study Knowledge   "Book Study" "Kingdom Hall"

I must pray morning, noon, & night.
Always ask God's help for a humble, spiritual attitude, & to rebuke the sexual feeling of fornication, jealously, & hatred.
I must ask God's help in providing me with patience for my son & etc.
And Jehovah God & Jesus Christ, I need your spiritual guidance to cover me & Jebdish, and help us to make the right decisions.
         In Jesus Christ Name, Amen.
I must stop spending money alone, and build a future for my son & I. Saving is the best policy.
Ask a trusted person for help. (Ruth & Annette)

(104)

Heart Broken Soulmate | 115

I wanna love you David. From your head to your toes. ♥

(76)

Why do I let people influence me, at times, to do something other than what my mind is made up to do??? For instance, I really wanted to move with my sister, so I won't be alone with Jediah, and have more help. Instead I stayed — because Burdell was home, just so he could leave again, and claim I've stranded in New Jersey. When I choose happiness, I never dreamed of having this lifestyle of loneliness, and unhappiness. I felt that if I had a kid, I would be married to the father. Getting married to Burdell, seems it will never be. It's not all about wearing a ring. It's about making that vow to God, stating your mate is the other half of you to make you One. Which it cuts away the sin of sexual relations if your not married. Marriage is making love with your mate, okay in God's Eye. Not being married is my major sin. I'm tired of having this sin attached to me. Before my Grandfather dies, I want him to be in my wedding.

110

Me ~~& You~~ Verse — Sketches from the Beggining

Love is in the air. Many lonely days & nights. But you came in my life. Letting me know my hopes & dreams will be. You are my inspiration, and friend. From beggining to end. Don't leave. So we can make love go futher.

I'm alone always. It's just my son and I. Being young, but I learned to survive on my own. I realize I can make it alone. Just my son & I can rely on each other. It's not so bad. We're already adjusted to the schedule. Of Surviving, Relying on God Almighty.

Everyday I go outside, brothers surprise me by saying I'm unique. Being alone with a son and looking nice. People watch me, as I come & go. I've never seen or payed any attention to the niggas outside. But different ones, new faces try to know me. They seem to know my neighbors, and I guess they tell them I live alone. Or don't have a boyfriend. I be nice, but tell all of them I'm spoken for. And they think I don't like them. I don't even know them. But like CeCe Penniston says: Keep On Walking. — That's what they need to see.

Dear Randell,

How are you? I'm doing okay, just gaining more weight. When I went to the doctor yesterday I now weigh 145 pounds. Aliyah's heartbeat is strong. Jerdiah is getting bigger & stronger by the day. He's very intelligent & smart. I called my health care, and they said my Lamaze Classes start July 12 - Aug 16th. Its a six week program, which is every Monday Eve 7pm - 9pm. At Norfolk General. They say I have to bring in my own couch. Do you want to be my partner? Yes or No. Anyway, I Love You, and wish you the best with your career. Keep your head up, and always pray to ask for Jehovah's Guidance, Protection, and Strength. I want to apologize for my behavior. I've been going through a ruff time dealing with working, taking care of Jerdiah, gaining weight, and my grandfather passing. My brain is going over 100 miles per hour, and at times I don't think before I speak. I thank you for your patience and always being there for me.

"Make Sure You Write Me Back"

Love Your Life,
Sonta

Time: 11:15 PM
Date: June 16th 1999
Mood: Relaxing

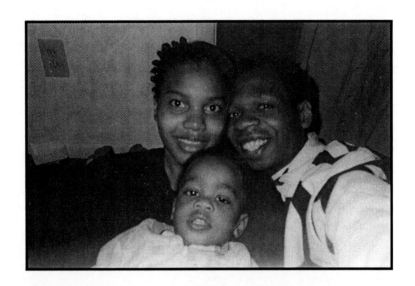

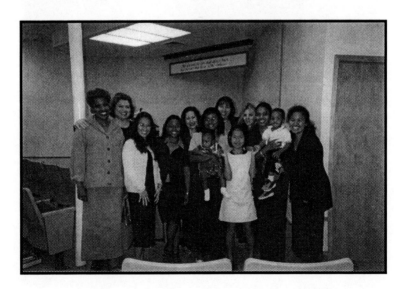

EIGHT
Third Child

MEANWHILE, BACK IN JERSEY I started hustling again so I could come home with some money.

My friend Cutter wanted to move down South where Vernon and I were.

Cutter was Vernon's younger cousin and he produce music.

Cutter ,David Glover, Hakeem, Darryle, Nicole, Dawoo, Sheryl, Ant and me would get up at Hakeem's house to get high and make songs all night long.

The following day, I went to my grandma's house.

She told me," Sonita called and said that, she was moving in with a friend.

She was tired of waiting for you so she's moving.

I said, "What?" I called to her grandfather's house, they haven't heard from her.

Nonetheless her grandfather ask me, "When are you coming back down here? You know she needs you." I told him, "I'm leaving this weekend."

I felt like I wasn't accomplishing anything up here.

I told Vernon, to send me my dough so I could leave.

He told me, "Help Cutter move down here, then I'll pay you."

So I did. Once we got to my house, Sonita wasn't there.

I was nervous and scared. I walked into the room it was clean.

I checked the bathroom, it was water inside the tub. I checked it.

The water was warm. I turned to Cutter and said, "She had to have just left. Let's go to the bus stop."

When we walked out of the door, she was coming down the street with Jehdiah.

She started smiling when she realized it was me, Jehdiah was trying to get out of the stroller.

I hugged her, and then I picked Jehdiah up. I introduced her to Cutter, then we went inside. I asked her, "Who is this person you are supposed to be moving in with?"

She gave me a smirk, and then said, "Your grandma told you about her?" I said, "Her, I thought it was a guy."

She said, "I knew you would, that's why I told your grandma a friend." I said, "That's a good one."

She smiled, and said, "It worked, you're here. She laughed.

I said, "You got that off. Is there anything to eat?" She said "No." I said, "Cutter before you turn in, take us to get something to eat." He did, and then he dropped us off.

We ate and I caught her up on all the things that happened.

We made love and fell to sleep.

I continued to work with Vernon, and Cutter joined in.

I went back to the barbershop part time and Sonita and I started attending the Kingdom Hall on the regular.

It was a happy time for us. We grew both closer to God and much closer to one another.

I caught us up on our bills and I had her on bed rest because she was getting bigger.

Jehdiah's first birthday came and Sonita invited a lot of people from her family to come.

She stayed up all night setting up. I helped her by making several trips to the store.

On the day of his birthday a majority of her family didn't show.

I was sitting on the couch, and she was in the kitchen telling me about all the people she had invited, and no one was there yet. I said,

"Well, our next door neighbors have children, we can invite them."
She slam the plate down and said,
"My family should be here! Its Jehdiah's first birthday."
Then, she started crying uncontrollably. She frightened Jehdiah and he ran to me.

I picked him up, walked over to her, and hugged her with Jehdiah in my arms. I said,
"We are here." Then, I put Jehdiah down as I hugged and kissed her.

I said, "Don't worry, somebody will come."
I really didn't know for sure, but I wanted to make her feel better.

I went next door, got the neighbor's children and I invited the adults over too.

I told them we could get our eat on and drink on then chill. I let the kids in, then I went to the store to get some beer. When I got back two cars were in my driveway.

I went inside to see her Aunt Annette, her brother Eric, and her twin cousins.

Sonita was happily smiling.

Annette bought Jehdiah a lot of toys while Eric got him a car.

Eric and I went outside so he could smoke. Sonita came outside and said she needed something else from the store, and her brother took me. We kicked it for a while about music, then he threw on an instrumental.

It was on from there. The adults from next door came over and we had a party!

Afterwards, everybody left and together we watch Jehdiah playing with his toys.

April rolled around and I turned 29. May came around and we were still going to the kingdom hall.

However, there were two certain elders who would always inquire about the date we were getting married.

I had already told them, several times, I had to get my divorce finalize first.

It seemed to us that, lately when we came, they would avoid talking to us.

We knew we were there for the message and not the people.

After a while, it discouraged Sonita, but I knew the truth; they were right. We couldn't make spiritual progress unless we separated, and served Jehovah in different places, until we were able to marry one another.

Sonita wasn't having that. She felt she had done the beginning of the year alone and she wasn't trying to be apart any longer.

June came around and we received a surprise visit from my brother, Ibn and Keisha.

They bought us food and played cards with us. We really had a nice time.

Sonita was kicking everybody's tail in Casino.

We were partners in Spades and they won 2 to 1.

Then my brother and I kicked it for awhile. After that, they broke out.

I had a court case for June in reference to my children.

Presently, I was working two jobs and I couldn't make it.

I wrote the courts, but I didn't get a response back.

After all that I went through, they granted custody to the aunt because I didn't show up.

It's been many times they didn't show up. They gave them continuances. First time I don't show, a decision is made. I was very very hurt over that.

However, I had my new family and I realized dejectedly that, I had to move on.

Work was slack with Vernon so I went fulltime in the shop.

I would cut hair from 9am to 9pm. Monday through Saturday.

Sonita hated those hours because by the time I got home I was too tired to talk.

I just wanted to sleep.

She wanted to tell me how her day had been. She told me she was in a lot of pain.

Her back was bothering her all the time, and I used to rub it for her. Then, I would give her a full body massage.

She quit working, which meant I had to step up.

I did, however she wanted me home earlier.

I explained that by doing this, I would lose out on money, although she wanted a change; she couldn't take it any more. She felt like I was staying longer hours in the shop because I had a girlfriend and didn't want to be bothered with her. Especially now that she's big, but that wasn't the truth.

I knew I couldn't manage the bills by leaving early. However, she wasn't having that.

Afterwards I started coming home early and the money decreased.

I began falling behind on bills, July rent was late, plus slacking at the meetings didn't make it any better.

Sonita came up with an idea.

She said, "My sister Kim said she would pay for me to come to Hawaii, and I could get myself together. Once you get your divorce, we could get married and serve Jehovah faithfully.

She can help me with Jehdiah; her son is a little younger than Jehdiah, so he will have a playmate." I said, "How long are you planning on being over there?"

She said, "How long will it take for you to get a divorce?"

I said, "No longer than six months to a year."

She said, "Well, I'll be in Hawaii serving Jehovah, while you serve him over here."

She continued, "I'm going to get my G.E.D, my license, plus save some money.

Our new child would only be about six months old and Jehdiah would be going on two.

Then we can reunite and get married. What do you think?"

I said, "Why do you have to go so far? I won't be able to see you period.

What's wrong with you just going to one of your family members' in the beach?"

She said, "Now you know that if we are close, we're going to continue to have sex."

I thought for a minute. She was right.

Using that time apart, I could get myself together with Jehovah and get my divorce.

I can prove to her that I do really want to marry her.

There was no doubt in my mind that I loved her and our son.

If she felt this was best, I told her, "You have my full support.

When do you plan on going?" She said, "In two weeks." I said, "Two weeks! The baby won't be born yet.

I want to see my son be born. Our last one died and I wasn't there. I want to see this one come out."

She said, "I'll send you some pictures." I said, "Pictures, I don't want to see no pictures! I want to see my baby!"

Then she said, "Just trust in Jehovah, he will make a way."

I said to myself, she using my words on me.

I said, "Okay." Then she said, "You're going to let me go?"

I said, "Yes, I'm going to put myself to the test and trust in Jehovah to guide us through."

We made love that night and afterwards she cried the hardest I had ever seen.

I didn't know what was wrong with her.

She kept saying, "I'm a miss you bay. Im a miss you."

I said, "We are going to get back together, right?" She said, "Yes." in a crying tone,

"But I love you so much. I don't think I can leave you?" I said, "Sonita I will be alright.

It will be the first time in ten years I'll be without any one to care for.

I promise you I'll get the divorce and serve Jehovah, plus I'll pay for you to come back, if you don't want to stay over there any longer."

I hugged and kissed her, then we fell asleep in each other's arms.

The next two weeks went by fast. Next thing I knew, we were on our way to the airport. That was the longest ride ever. Once we arrived, we slowly went to the floor the plane was leaving on.

We both cried, hugged, kissed and said goodbye.

The only thing I knew was that my soulmate is now in the sky.

I was crushed and hurt. I said to myself, I'm a trust in you Jehovah, because I know you can oversee our plans and help us accomplish our goals.

Then I said to myself, someone will be loving my girl, she is too pretty not to have someone. I just pray she doesn't get strung out over him and don't come back. Knowing me, I'll go over there and get her.

Then, I immediately rejected the thought and said, "Jehovah please help me."

I stayed there until I couldn't see the plane any more. Then I bounced and went to work.

It was the hardest and longest day of my life. Everyone who came in knew something was wrong. I tried to hide my hurt, but it was evident. I shut the shop down at 10:00pm that night. I stayed in the shop because I didn't have a phone at home. I called Sonita to make sure she got there safely. Her sister answered the phone and said, "Damn she hasn't got here yet and you are already calling?"

I said, "Dig Kim, that's my girl and children on the airplane. I want to know if they made it, period." Kim said, "I apologize for that Randell. They haven't gotten here yet, it was a two hour lay over in California. When she gets here, I'll have her call you."

I said, Thank you. Then I hung up.

I work the next day and she calls me. We talked for a while, then I talked to Jehdiah.

I felt much better. Mohammed got a hair cut, then he took me home.

My house felt so empty, I didn't know what to do.

Now I actually knew how Sonita felt now that she was gone.

I was bored and I didn't know what to do with myself. I got on my knees and prayed to Jehovah for help to get through this day. I was in tears.

After that, I read the Bible. Then I wrote Sonita a letter. Finally, I took it down and fell asleep. We talked on the phone everyday for two weeks, then I received a letter from her.

The letter moved me because I could tell she was at peace. She had no worries, because her sister Kim is looking out for her. She can concentrate on her goals, and really be all she could be. She told me about two Jehovah Witnesses she met, they were her age and they were baptized. They used to take her around the Island and she really enjoyed serving Jehovah.

Then on August 31,1999 her water broke, and her sister took her to the hospital.

She called me and told me it was time. I told her to have Kim call me after you have the baby. Kim called me three hours later and said she had him. He was a big baby, and they took pictures. I was so happy that Abijah was healthy and vibrant, that I ran out my house screaming," I have a son, I have a son!" I called Jazz, Teric, and Samad. They congratulated me. Then Samad said, "Yo I'm on my way, so we can celebrate."

Consequently, it dawned on me, Abijah was born on the same day my mother died.

How Ironic is that. I immediately made it up in my mind to stop doing drugs and stop drinking. I wanted to serve Jehovah right. I smoked and drank my last beer September 12,1999. In the meantime, Sonita and I stayed in touch. She kept me informed on the children. If she needed anything for them I would send it. I made progress quickly and before long I was an unbaptized publisher. I wrote Sonita every week, but she would just call me back. Finally after me complaining about wanting a letter she wrote me again.

Dear Randell,   August 11, 1999
                                            At 4:30 am.

    I love you baby. I always will. We've been through alot. Many good and bad times. We've shared the joy of having 3 beautiful little boys, Jehdiah, Josiah, and Abijah. I've been through alot. It's time I change my life's pattern, and do my best to make it into God's Kingdom. Jehdiah and Abijah depend on me to provide them the proper love, care, and spiritual teaching. Satan is very busy, because he has a short time. Everything happens for a reason. God is making a way for my kids and I to move to a better environment. He's relieving alot of stress I've been carrying for years. My mind is at peace, and I finally have happiness. We have alot of history. I appreciate all the help you've given me since I met you. I wish you the best, and pray that you recieve the peace and happiness you deserve. I hope you make it into God's Organization. Soon, you won't have to worry about bills, money, sickness, violence, not seeing your kids. All the evil destructions Satan threw in your life will be no more. Serve Jehovah & Jesus Christ Baby. And you'll see him bless you with things you never thought you'll have. I Love You Randell. I will be your friend & family forever. Our kids Jehdiah, Abijah and myself will keep you in our prayers. We'll never forget you.   Love Your True Family
                                    (+Josiah+) Juanita, Jehdiah, & Abijah

Dear Randell,   1st Letter   (Date Written Tuesday) — Date Mailed —
                                                        August 24, 1999

I miss you so much. Jerdiah looks more like you everyday. I hug & kiss him more, because he reminds me of you. I always knew how much love I have for you. I feel it more from the distance. Knowing you're so far, hurts. I feel alone. I look forward to us reuniting. I'm on a mission to keep my time occupied. I have no excuse to not have my life in harmony with Jehovah & Jesus Christ.

Here Is A List Of My Goals:
- Serve Jehovah & Jesus Christ
- Teach Jerdiah & Alijah, so they can grow up pleasing God / And Always Do What's Right
- Attend All meetings at the Kingdom Hall
- Work on my personality, attitude. AND OTHER THINGS THAT MAKE YOU Fall
- Get G.E.D.
- Get License
- Get A Job
- Work On Saving Money ** FOR WHEN TIMES GET FUNNY **
- Pay Back Overdue Bills
- Work on Getting A Car TO BUILD
- Get My Own Apartment LOVE LIFE AND KEEP IT REAL
- Keep Putting Jehovah & Jesus Christ First In My Life.

My Adrenalin is running, and my mind is made up. Jah is my first priority. He has to be. That's the only way doors of success can be open for me. I want to live to see paradise on Earth. I want to hold my baby Josiah Again. And introduce him to Jerdiah & Alijah. Maybe even meet my mother & see your Mother Mardette. To Be Apart of a world full of Brothers & Sisters who love God with all their heart. I want to know God so my love for him will over-shadow me, and I'll Shine. I have so much Peace where I'm At. I'm sticking to my plan so my goals won't fail. Jerdiah Misses You. He touch your picture and say Da Da. Then he holds his right hand up and talk to me while he touch your face. I think his fussing at me saying take me to Da Da. M. You know I Love & Miss Him. Keep Me In Your Prayers. Satan Is Busy. But I'm going to fight hard with the help of God. I Love You Randell. I'm grateful to have you as a friend & "In my Life." It was time for us to be apart, so He can Do What's Right. You can accomplish your goals without worrying about any distractions I've caused you. I'm safe Baby. Jah is Protecting Me and making a way for Jerdiah, Alijah, and I to make it. That's Why He Made a Way for me to move to a beautiful island, to give me a taste of what Paradise would be like. And he rescued me from the Death Trap Satan Had prepared for me in Norfolk. All those Bad Vibes I had are Gone. I Want you to make it Baby. Stay in the Kingdom Hall & Get Baptized. Put Jehovah and Jesus Christ First in your Life. I Love You Baby. Stay Safe.

Dear Randell;   2nd Letter   Date Written- Sunday Night 22nd.

I Love You. Everything is fine with Jehdiah & I. I took him to Emergency Thursday 19th. His temperature was 103.8. He has an ear infection. He's much better now. I make sure he takes his medication on time and drink plenty of fluids. That's my sweetheart. I'm so attached to Jehdiah & proud of him. He's the joy of my life and very smart. What's been up with you? "Are you making all your meetings Despite the time you attempted to go, But no-one was there."? I kept calling the Hall. A guy named Eddie answered the phone. I haven't met him yet. But he told me a sister will get in contact with me and help me with transportation arrangements. Her name is Mara Higo. She's Phillipino. Her Husband Randy is Japenise. I went to the book study Friday 20th, & the Meeting Sunday 22nd. I comment at the book study. Here in the Greatest Man Book Chapter 58, 59. Next Friday will be 61, 62, 63. I didn't comment # on Sunday's Meeting. I'll work on that next time. There's one other Black Women at the Hall. Everyone else is Phillipino, Japenise, Hawaiian, or White. But everyone I meet is very friendly, & Loving. They make Jehdiah & I feel very welcome.
My sister shows me alot of love. She say she's not against me attending the Hall, and never say anything bad about it. She told me she'll support whatever decision I make in my life. We're adjusting OKAY. I feel welcome at my sister's home. We been to two Malls. Both are very Nice with alot of activity insides. And I've also been to Waikiki Beach. For as far Back you can see, the water is a pretty light Blue. When I have Elijah & My schedule allow, I'll relax on the Beach more often. And take pictures so I can show you How it Look Out Here and where I Live. There's alot of Mountains. And People Have Homes on the mountains. It look like Jerusalem. And Villeys. Like at the bottom in between 2 Mountains is alot of Little Houses. The # Whole Senery out Here is nothing I wouldve ever imagine. I'm learning my way around everyday. I haven't been to the other islands yet. Yes it took me 16 hrs to get here on plane. I Left 1:00 pm. and got to Atlanta Georgia. 2:20 pm. (1 hr delay.) That's when I called you from that Airport. We left 3:40 pm. I got to California at 6:30 pm. But Note. Every certain distance, 1 hr. goes back. We had a 2 hr. Delay in San Francisco, California. The Plane had a Fuel Problem which scared me. From California to Hawaii Crossing the water alone is 5 hrs.

That's my long term Flying Experience. I don't ever want to Fly again. I can't wait to see you. Remember we have 6 months to accomplish our goals. Be careful when you go anywhere. And don't surround yourself with ungodly People. I Love You. Stay Safe. Can't Wait to See You But it's going to be Much Love When we Meet Again.

Your Future Wife Sonita.

P.S. No I don't have men trying to get with me. I'm strictly attending the Hall and doing Whats Right. Are You Doing the Same???

Write Me Back Soon !!!

Remember My Due Date is Aug 24th.

2nd Letter

Jehdiah & I Love You Baby.
Abijah Does Too.

Dear Randell,   Sept 13, 1999
                                                                 Date Sent: Sept 16th

I Love You Baby. Be safe always, and pay close attention to your environment. (Revelation 12:9-12) Woe for the earth... because the Devil has come down to you, having great anger, knowing he has a short period of time. Never let Satan bring you down. Always Please Jehovah & Jesus Christ. God's Word foretold that in these last days, humble ones would be gathered together in a Global Society based on Love & Humility. Thus in the midst of a world that is becoming more and more prideful, Jehovah's People display the opposite attitude — lowliness of mind. God's Spirit working through his willing people enables them to learn to conquer the bad spirit of the world and then to demonstrate the fruitage of God's Spirit. This manifests itself in "love, joy, peace, long-suffering, kindness, goodness, faith, mildness, self-control". (Galatians 5:22,23). I learn alot from the Watch Tower August 1, 1999 — "Mind Yourselves With 'Lowliness of Mind'". I went to the Kingdom Hall Today. Well, actually I'm a regular attendant of all the Meetings. Alot of issues were discuss that I applied to myself. Reading this particular article open my eyes to alot of things. I'm eager to learn more about Jehovah & Jesus Christ. I feel very welcome in Hawaii. My home is Peaceful, and the Kingdom Hall refreshes me and my Spirit. I attend the Salt Lake Congregation. Adelle is my transportation to the meeting. She's 25 years old, already baptized, and very nice. She's going to come to my home every week, Here studying "What Does God Require From Us". She's helping me to build my knowledge, so I can go to the Theocratic Ministry School. Many doors of opportunity is opening for me. Everything is Great For Me. Jerdiah & Alijah is doing Excellent. My Sons are the joy of my life. I want to reside in Hawaii for good, and continue the good life I finally have. This is the best I've ever felt in my whole life. I know the last time I spoke to you, I did another 360. I'm becoming more spiritual and do more in my heart. I just wanted to share with you how I feel and give you an update on How things are going for me. But enough about me. I hope you ("enjoy & like") the pictures. Please send me some pictures, call and write me soon!!!!! Have a very Lovely Day, and Stay Spiritually Focused. It's the only way you can survive. Just focus on "always" doing what is right, and Please Jehovah & Jesus Christ. "Write Back Randell !!!" (P.S. I start school Sept. 27th.)

                                                            Love Always,
                                                            Sonita
                                                            Jerdiah & Alijah & Josiah

Dear Randell,   Wed. Sept. 15th 1999
                                                 Date Sent: Thurs. 16th.

How are you? I miss you! Your sons love & miss you too. I hope your doing okay. Be safe always & stop going outside after dark. Right now, the kids & I are downstairs. All of the upstairs area still smell like paint. I don't want Alijah & Jehdiah to inhale the fumes. David just bought me the envelope so I can send this package off tomorrow. "Finally"!!! It's 11:00 pm. The Chris Rock Show just came on. I'm not tired but I want to talk to you. I know it's 5:00 am where you're at. So I'll let you sleep. I wish we were together. We can prepare for the meeting together. And I would still beat you in Casino. If you forgot my skills, ask your brother Ibn. When you speak to Ibn tell him I asked about him and send him a picture of Alijah. I have a coupon for a free 8x10 photo at Sears. Jehdiah, Alijah, and I have to take pictures before the 30th of Sept. That's when the coupon expires. Well, I'll bring closure to this letter. I just want you to know I'm thinking of you. Alijah is beside me doing push-ups. He's up for the night. Jehdiah is sleep. Write Me Back!!!
Tell Christy & Katrina I said Hi!
                                                 Love You.
                                                 Sonita

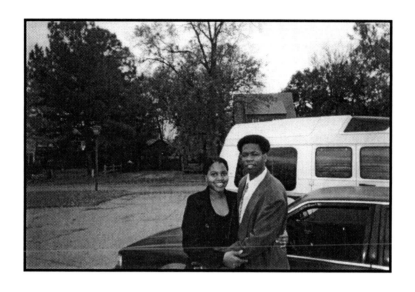

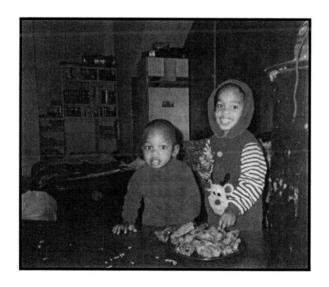

NINE
Spiritual Test

I CONTINUED TO GO to the Kingdom Hall and out in field service.

People who came to my job saw a change in me.

I would play Bible tapes with drama stories about Noah, Moses, and Joshua. I had the Watch Towers and Awake Magazines on display, as well as the regular Jet, Ebony, Source, and Vibe Magazines. I had pictures up of my family and I would witness to whoever was interested. I felt Jehovah's presence in my life. I was very happy. I just missed my family a lot. However, I knew I would reunite with them one day.

I talked to Sonita on the phone and she sounded different. She just went off on me. I was confused. I said," Why are you mad at me, I didn't do nothing?"

Sonita said," In the past you did and I don't want to be bothered with you any more."

I thought to myself. She met somebody over there and now she is flipping on me.

I said, "Who is he?"

She said, "Why do you think it's somebody?"

I said, "I just talked to you a week ago and you were fine, now you are flipping on me because of our past? Sounds like to me you are trying to find an excuse to break up with me."

She said," We are friends and I can do what I want."

I said, "Who are you hanging out with?"

She said, "My cousins, why?"

I said, "I knew it couldn't be any Jehovah Witnesses because you wouldn't be talking to me like this."

She said, "Whatever." Then she hung up on me.

I was hurt but I knew it was destined to happen. She is beautiful inside and out.

You rarely find that in a pretty woman. Now I had to prepare myself for whatever goes down. I went out in field service the following morning with Brother and Sister Young.

I told her about our conversation, and that I was going over there to check up on her.

She said, "Don't do that."

I said, "Why?"

She said, "Because Sonita has to learn on her own to trust in Jehovah and have faith.

It's easy for her to depend on you or her sister because she can see ya'll, however, she has to learn how to trust in God; who she can't see."

I said, "But she is slipping."

Then Sister Johnson said, "I know it's a part of the process."

I said," Process, what do you mean?"

She continued, "I'll give you an example. My husband and me for instance; when we started serving Jehovah, the Devil worked on the weaker one out of the two to break up both of us and get us off track. I was doing good, but my husband was doing bad.

I couldn't give up on Jehovah or him. I had to stick with Jehovah regardless of what he took me through. That way I build up my faith on my own. I had to trust in Jehovah to bring my husband around."

I said, "So, you mean she's probably going to do things she normally wouldn't because of the devil's influence over her?"

She said, "Yep."

Then I said, "Ill. I have to be the stronger one in order to put up with it and show through my faithfulness. She could do the same?"

She said, "Yes"

Then I said, "Well, that's another reason why I should go over there."

Mrs. Johnson said, "No, you shouldn't, because you will discourage her with your progress, instead of encouraging her."

I said, "Wow I just got to deal with it and stay faithful to Jehovah."

She said, "Yes, all couples who are trying to serve Jehovah go through it."

I concluded with," Thanks for that insight, but what can I do from here?"

Mrs. Johnson smiled and said, "Keep writing and encouraging her. Let her know, you understand and only want the best for her. Also, you are proud of her for even trying to serve God. Persevere in prayer."

I was grateful for that information. I stayed out in field service for about two hours then I went home, changed and bounced to work. I called Sonita later on that day.

She sounded much better than before. After our conversation, I cut hair for the rest of the day witnessing between clients. Sabrina came by the shop and chilled with me.

I liked her because she was different from the other girls who liked me. I could talk to her about Sonita and ask her question about women and she would tell me. She had two beautiful daughters, one 4 and the other 1 year old. Sometimes on my way home I would stop by her house and talk with her before my bus came to take me home. She was a single parent raising her two girls by herself. Their fathers were locked up.

It seemed like every time we were about to get intimate, Sonita would page me and I'd be scared to death. I would leave and call her. Sonita would say something like," You were on my mind." To me, I took it as a sign not to allow our relationship to go any further than a friendship. Plus, Satan always sets his trap for whenever I was feeling down lonely or stressed out. I would go home and pray to Jehovah. When I would awake in the morning, I felt so good to know that I didn't give in. October came around and Sonita told me she wanted to go into the Air Force. I said,

"What!"

She said, "I will be able to get benefits from the military to help me in college and travel the world." I said, "And where are my children going to be?"

She explained that her sister will have them. I said, "No, she is not. It's no way I'm going to allow my sons to be without me because of your decision to sign your life away. If you want to go, my sons are gonna be with me. Anyway Jehovah doesn't approve of us taking up arms to kill people. Jesus Christ said for us to remain separate from the world, just like he was. Can you picture Jesus Christ in an airplane fighting for the president of the United States?" (John 17:14-16, John 18:36-37.)

She laughed and said, "No, but I need security." I said "You can get that from Jehovah."

She exclaimed, "See you never support my decision, that's why we are growing a part."

Then she hung up. I thought for a minute, someone is filling her head with this mess.

I called back and she didn't want to talk to me so she hung up on me again!

I was pissed off. I knew she was doing this because she knew I couldn't get to her.

I finished cutting and my clients could see something was bothering me, but only Alicia asked me what was wrong. She was a girl who use to live in my hometown. We met down here in the barbershop, I cut her son's hair. We got along fine, however I didn't know her that well to tell her my business. I told her, "I'm tired that's all."

She said, "No your not, you are stressing over that girl in Hawaii."

I said, "How did you figure that?"

She continued, "Because, when you are in a good mood you're usually reading the Bible or talking about God. Now you're quiet."

I said," Well, you're right it's Sonita, but I'll deal with it. Thanks for your concern; however I'd rather not talk about it." After I cut her son's head I left and went home.

Once I got there, I cried like a baby. I felt it in my heart that I was slowly losing her.

We barely talked for the next two weeks. Shockingly she called me out of the blue.

She said, "I'm sorry for the way I was acting towards you. I really miss you Randell, and the boys do too."

I told her the same; then I shared with her how my day had gone out in field service.

I asked her about school and the meeting.

Sonita said," The teachers are prejudiced towards people from the mainland, which means the U.S. they feel like we come over here and take the good jobs from them."

She continued, I'm still going to the Kingdom Hall, but it something I want to ask you."

I said, "What?"

She said, "Would you mind if I go to a party with my cousin?"

I said, "What kind of party?"

She said, "A Halloween party, but it's not on Halloween."

I said, "What difference does it make? It's still a party glorifying the devil and demons.

I can't go for that."

She spoke softly and said, "I don't go anywhere, plus I want to go out with my cousin."

Then I thought for a minute. She really loves and respect me because she didn't have to ask or tell me. I said, "You know the truth, so there's no need to ask me, just take it up with God. Me myself I wouldn't go."

Then she said, "Will you be mad?"

I said, "No, that's your decision, you have to answer to God the same way I do; just be safe and careful."

Then she said, "I will here is my cousin who's taking me." I talked to him for a minute.

I told him," Take care of my girl." He said, "She will be fine." Then he gave her back the phone.

Sonita said, "I don't know for sure if I'm going, but I'll talk to you tomorrow."

Meanwhile, I continued to work and later I went to the meeting. The next day she called and told me she went and had fun. I was happy that she had gone out; however, I felt sad that she's easily influenced. But, then again, she never partied before. She is experiencing life now. I did it when I was her age, so I couldn't fault her.

I would just write her three letters a week and encourage her to stay focused.

I knew it had to be hard to do. She was in paradise. A happy, fun island with partying going on everywhere.

November came around and she told me she changed her mind about the Air Force. The sister who studied with her came over with the latest Watch Tower and Awake Magazines. The Awake talked about the military and our neutral stand as disciples of Jesus Christ.

I was happy to hear that, however, it bothered me because when I told her, she said I wasn't supportive; then a sister shows her and she listened. Then I took it as my prayers were answered, and I knew Jehovah was helping us both individually. I was running through calling card after calling card, so I asked her to start back writing me.

She hadn't written me since September. She received three letters a week from me, all the way to November.

She felt kind of bad about it, so she wrote me after I had sent off a package for her. It had kid's clothes, pictures, diapers, letters, a money order, and a slow jam tape which I made for her.

Dear Randell, — From Sonita, Jehdiah, and Abijah

Saturday Nov. 13, 1999
Mood - Relaxed.
2:30 AM Good Morning
Just Finish Taking A Shower
And Washing Jehdiah.
He's Falling Asleep
Abijah is Sleep!
I Got Your Package
Tonight
Friday 12th.
I'm Listening
to your tape
Now! !!!

Hi Baby! I hope you're doing well. I Apologize for taking so long to right you back. My days go by so quickly. Your letter was uplifting for me; and I appreciate you taking the time out of your busy schedule, to share with me your wisdom. I'm doing the count down for my N.E.D. Test December 6, 7, & 8. I'm very nervous. Today I sent my entry in for The Best of Rap City CD Contest. All you do is write the songs in the order they play them.; And you can win $20,000. I wish I win because that cash would be a big help. Abijah is getting huge. He's my sweet chocolate baby. His complexion is between mine and yours. When I take some more pictures, I'll send them to you. Jehdiah is getting tall. He's my heart. Out of the blue, I ask Jehdiah "Where Is Your Teeth, Nose, & Eyes"? He pointed to each. He know his hands and feet also. He grew so fast. It still feels like yesterday when I gave birth to him. I was so excited & happy. Now my baby is repeating words he hear. "Juice, Eat Eat, Ma Ma, Baby, Hi, Bye Bye, No, What are you talking about?"; everything else he say is Phillipino Language. Well Randell, I still Love You. And I love the beautiful cards, letters, Watch Tower Pictures, and tapes you sent me. You really Brighten my Day, and made me feel good. Also, If "You" feel like nobody loves or care about you, Always "Remember" Jehovah and Jesus Christ Does! (Always Smile!! Bye!!)

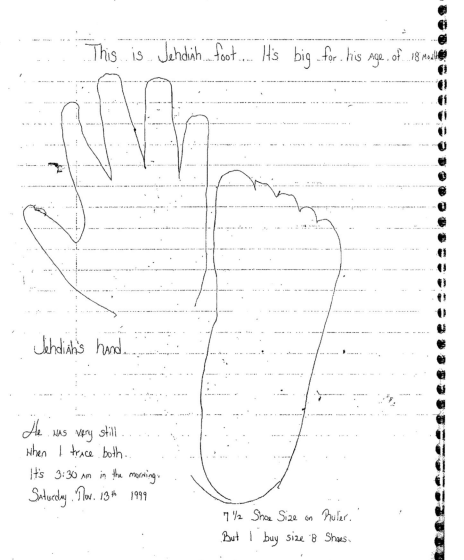

Randell, This is how big Abijah foot is. He WAS sleep when I trace this. He has big feet for 2½ months of age. He kept moving his foot. I think I was tickling him.

(It's 9:15 am.)
Saturday Nov. 13th 1999

This is Abijah's Hand. He kept taking his hand away from me. Now he's awake.

133.

I read her letter and it was very uplifting. I could see she still loved me but, I still felt in my heart, she was seeing someone else.

Our conversations from that point on were strictly about the children. If I talked about us she would catch an attitude. Her conversations were mainly about school and hanging out with her cousin. I couldn't blame her for that. He was her family and they would have fun together. I still stuck to the plan. I filed for my divorce from Susan. I worked and went to the Kingdom Hall. I saved money. As a matter of fact, this was the most money I had ever made cutting hair down in V.A. I owed it all to Jehovah.

I went to the Kingdom Hall and a Sister asked me, if I wanted to buy her car.

I said," What kind?"

She told me a Hyundai. I told her," Yes, let me check it out." I did and it was better than the Chevrolet I bought from my neighbor. I figured, I'll buy it for Sonita for when she comes back. I told Sonita about it and she told me not to buy it for her because she wasn't coming back to V.A.

My heart was crushed; I felt the lump in my throat. I couldn't even think straight.

I went home early from the shop and cried myself to sleep. Even though each week there was something brand new going on with Sonita, I was happy to be doing Jehovah's Will.

I wasn't drinking, getting high or having sex. I had a good conscience. I knew at this point that if I died, Jehovah would resurrect me in paradise right here on earth.

But in the meantime, I was lonely as ever once I got home. I moved out of Ocean view to Little Creek Road into a studio apartment. It was only me therefore it was no need to keep the two bedroom; besides she said she wasn't coming back. I figured once my divorce was final, I'd go to Hawaii to get her. December came around and I was still on schedule. A number of girls were coming by the shop, and they were looking good.

They all wanted me, but I couldn't do it. I haven't been this close to Jehovah in years and it felt great! On the down side, I was so far from the love of my life and I was so incomplete without my family. I couldn't see my four children in Brooklyn, my other son who was in Irvington New Jersey or my two sons in Hawaii. I put together a video tape of me talking to her and I was planning on sending it right before I came to Hawaii.

Sonita calls and tell me her Aunt Annette came out there to visit. They all went to the beach together. Her sister's friend was selling her a car in order for her to get around. I just listened because I couldn't say anything about us because she would get mad and hang up on me. A couple of days later, she tells me she's sorry. I just prayed and prayed for us. Finally, she calls me and say," If I come back, can we move to Atlanta; I heard its a Black Mecca. We can do good down there. Randell, I really don't want to come back to V.A." I said, "I can check it out. I'm tired of being here too, especially without you."

Sonita said," Why do you put up with me?"

I said, "Because I love you for real. You are my heart. And this time apart has proven it to me. I know I haven't been the best man in the past, but with Jehovah, we can have a better future. Matter of fact, I'll pay for ya'll to come back. She said, "When?"

I said, "When you're ready; I'm more stable now. I have two cars, a place to stay and God by my side. We can make it. All we have to do is start fresh from the time you get back, okay?"

She said, "Okay."

I can't lie though, it was getting the best of me; tearing me apart inside and out. I was so stressed that I started back writing in my diary.

my diary

Feb 2, ???

① I got up this morning and I prayed to Jehovah. Then I studied the daily text. Afterward I layed out the plan to make sure I send the money order back to the Dentist company. And call Bro Blunt so I can get my life insurance. After I call Pam and told her I mailed the money order. I call Bro Blunt he said we will hook up today. Then I went to the travel agent to get my money back plus make the change on the ticket. Karen wasn't there so I went to work. I studied the lessons that was going to be discuss tonight in the Kingdom Hall. Then I started cutting. Afterwards I went back to see Karen. And she was there. We talk about the price range and it was high!!! She told me she would try to work with the days to see if she can get it cheaper. I said O.K. fine. Then I left and went to the Health department so I can take the T.B. test. That way I can start the substituting job.

Randell Barkley
Life in the year 2000

The beggining of this year January 1 2000 I was alone. And throughout this month I've been tempted by woman almost every day to have sex. Or go out with them didth I've been making my meetings and I've been going out on field service. I've been struggling with a masterbation habit that has slowed down greatly but hasn't stop completly. My baby mother Sonita has told me she left V.A. for a reason, and shes "moving on". I ask her who is he? She told me its non of my business who she talk to I told her I was coming to Hawaii. She told me not to come. I ask her is you my girl? She said not right now!!

I cried many nights because of our conversation and prayed very hard for answers. And through all of this I will not leave my GOD Jehovah and I have not kiss or had sex with any women still

now its the month of February

The next day was the second part of questions for baptism. When Brother Copo arrived, he could see in my face I wasn't feeling to good. He asked me what was wrong and I broke out in tears and told him everything that happened. I felt terrible and worthless. This was the closest I've ever been towards getting Baptized and I blew it.

He encouraged me to continue attending the meetings and go out in field service.

He helped me appreciate that I couldn't give up. I'm only human, so I must rely soley on Jehovah for strength to overcome my weakness because I can't do it on my own.

I'm not a lost cause. Jehovah is merciful and ready to forgive as long as we repent and work hard at not doing it again. I realized something. Sonita had my mind and heart. Whatever she does affected me. I can't allow her to break me, so I went to work and tried to stay optimistic. I continued to preach to people even though I was hurting inside.

The next day was February 13, 2000 and I went out in field service with Brother Cook, and Brother Owings. They encouraged me not to give up on God. They really brightened up my day. They dropped me off at work and my cousin Jazz called me.

He told me he thought he was gonna die because his blood pressure shot up and he was in critical condition all week.

He would've been dead a week now.

He lost a kidney and was on dialysis for six years now. We talked on the phone for about a hour and I cheered him up.

Sabrina came in the shop with her two girls. She informed me, that she broke up with her baby daddy. He had some other girl visiting him and Sabrina found out.

I thought to my self, the devil is busy! I'm here trying to convince Sabrina to stay with her man and my girl just dumped me for another dude. I've been depressed all week. I haven't eaten in 5 days and my body is in severe pain. I don't want to be at work.

I told Sabrina, that Sonita dumped me and everything. She suggested we go get something to eat at Alices. I was with that.

Once we arrived there, my pager went off and it was Sonita! I was shocked because it was 9am over there. She never called me that early. I told Sabrina, "Never mind the food, I got to go call Sonita."

Sabrina screamed out," Now Love, you need to eat first, make her wait. You look defeated. Eat something!"

I said," I'm, I'm cool. I'll be alright, I'm not that hungry any way." Then I started walking away. Sabrina grabbed my arm and said," It's a shame how much that girl got your mind; you gonna starve yourself just to talk to her. Come over my house later and I'll cook for you." She let me go and walked away. I went to 7 Eleven and called her.

I said, "What's up Sonita?"

She said," Oh I just want to come clean with you, I've been talking to my cousin's friend and we like each other. He told me I was one of a kind."

I said," And you fell for that? I used to say the same line, I can't believe it still works."

She continued," Well he wants me to move in with him. He has a nice place and a car."

I said, "So do I, but never mind that; if you want to be with him go ahead; but my sons are not going to be without me. So you got a choice, either bring them to me or I'm coming over there to be with them. You can have them for 6 months out the year and I'll have them for the other 6 months; that way you and your friend can be together."

I really didn't mean what I was saying, but I didn't want her to hear me upset or crying like I was inside.

I further told her," If you want to go backwards with someone you barely know, instead of going forward with me and get married in two months. Go right ahead, I'm sticking with Jehovah. You can live in sin with him, however I wont allow you to drag my sons down with you. I'm going to be in their life."

Sonita paused for a moment, then she said," I can't believe I'm having this conversation with you, I'm crazy right?"

I said," You said it not me."

She concluded with, "Well I just wanted to tell you what was really going on; I feel you deserve to know. I'll call you back later with what I'm going to do."

I said, "Okay." Then I hung up. I walked back to the shop heartbroken, with a headache, stomachache, back pains, dehydrated, pissed off, upset, mad, hurt, and hungry!!

I worked half the day and went home and cried myself to sleep.

A week later, I get a letter from her.....

TEN
Marriage

Now it was all in the open. I told her, "I slept with a total stranger that night you came clean with me about you sleeping with old dude.

Being that I hadn't remained faithful to Jehovah like I should, I fell into pieces.

I won't be getting baptized this assembly.

I have to wait another six months before I can requalify."

She said, "For real Love? Well, I don't want you out late after work. Go straight home and don't be giving those heifers my loving. By the way, did you go down on her?" I said,

"Hell No!" I'm not infatuated like you.

I did it out of spite, being hurt, and not spiritually strong enough to endure. I don't ever want to do that again. I want to marry you, but you are involved with someone else." She said,

"That's not for long Bay, I'm coming home to you.

I want to be your wife." I excitedly asked,

"Really?" She lovingly responded,

"Yes, Love, really." At that moment I said,

"Well, when you get back our life together will start then.

What we did before we reunited, is not going to be held against us." She paused for a minute and said,

"Okay Love, I'm with that."

Then we hung up.

I didn't know if I was coming or going. The only thing I was trying to maintain was my meeting attendances at the Kingdom Hall.

A week goes by, then I get a call. It was Sonita saying,

"Look, Love, I changed my mind. I want to live over here."

I said, "Well I'm coming out there to see you and my sons!"

She asked, "For what? I don't want you to come out here."

I told her, "Now you're bugging, I'll see you soon;"

Then I hung up.

Sonita called me right back.

However, I wouldn't answer the phone.

It rang four times and each time she hung up on the ninth ring.

I left work and walked down to the Travel Agent's place on Colley avenue, across from Blair Middle School.

The lady was very nice and warm towards me.

I told her where I was going and she tried to help me get the best rate.

Sonita had my mind. I mean total control of my mind and she was so far away. I had to see her face to face to know whether our love was real. My whole life was hanging in the balance awaiting her decision. The cost was high, but I was willing to sacrifice my money and time to see my sons and her. I haven't seen my other children from my first wife since '98, and it's 2000. Sonita is being influenced by some dude to keep my children away from me. I called and doubled up on sending my letters to her. However, she didn't want to talk to me. Our conversations were real short. I asked her if she read any of the letters I sent her and she told me no.

Then, I realized she was trying to get me out her system.

All I could do was rely on Jehovah to help me.

Another Idea came to my mind. I'll make her a video tape and send it to her. She can watch it along with my children. Hopefully, she can see the sincerity in my plea to bring my children back to me. I made it in one week. The day I plan to send it, I get a call from Sonita. She tells me, "I'm coming back home. I don't want to stay here."

I asked her, "Why?" She replied,

"My sister is leaving the Island in October of this year, plus my cousin is going to Korea in June. None of my family will be over here. I'll be stuck with my friend and I don't trust him like that." I said,

"Word? Well, when are you trying to come back?"

She said, "In June sometime." I said,

"Hell no! I want to see my sons before that. I'll pay for ya'll to come back.

You already have your G.E.D., your license and money saved. Come home now, why waste time?" She said,

"Love, I don't want to come back and struggle.

That's all we seem to do." I said,

"Its different now, I'm not struggling. Jehovah blessed me and he's guiding me. I have two cars, an apartment, plus I've been saving money." She said,

"I'll come in April so we can be together.

What's the deal with your divorce? I told her,

"It should be coming through real soon.

I'll go back to the travel agent and see how much it will cost me to bring ya'll all back. I'll talk to you in a couple of days."

Tuesday I went and priced it at the Travel Agency. The cheapest I could find was $1,687.00 for all of them. Cindy could see by my reaction, it was out of my range. I would definitely be cutting into my savings.

She suggested I go online to cheap tickets.com to see if I could get a cheaper price.

I called Sonita to tell her what happened and she sounded down.

I said, "What's wrong, baby you don't sound right?" She said,

"I know, I'm just tired and confused." I replied with,

"Confused about what?" She responded,

"If it's really gonna work." I told her,

"Well, Sonita, the only thing I can say is, I'm going to put my trust in God to make it work. Just leave it in his hands and be real with yourself." She said,

"Maybe, I need to stay a little longer to save more money."

I said, "Sonita you should go back to the meetings so you can feel better; learn some things you know." She said,

"Okay Bay; what's up, why did you call?" I said,

"I want to tell you it's gonna cost me about $1,600.00 to get ya'll back, but I'm a see if I can get it cheaper through the internet.

Now, when I get the tickets, I'll send it to you; make sure you're on that plane!" She said excitedly,

"I will, I will."

The next day is Wednesday; I pay for my divorce then I went to the library to get on the internet. The lady there was very patient and understanding with me, because I didn't know how to get to the site. We shopped for the lowest prices between $1,680.00 to $2,056.00 On the third of April it cost $1,687.00 If they leave on the fourth it's $1,368.00 My goal is to meet the $1,368.00

They gave me a 1-800 number. I left and went back to the barbershop. The first thing that came to my mind was, my rent is due, which is $420.00

My booth rent is $75.00 I figure I get $300.00 from Sonita and the ticket will be bought. I just paid $90.00 for my divorce.

Now, all together, it's $1,953.00 I need to cover in this week.

After spending $90.00 that left me with $810.00

I'm cutting hair in the barbershop, then I throw on one of my Bible tapes.

I see people reading magazines, but they are listening.

Afterwards, I throw on a love tape. The whole time I'm thinking about my family. Around 3 O'clock, in the afternoon, I got a break so I called up 1-800 cheap tickets. The man said,

"April the fourth is booked, can she leave another day?"

I said, "Yeah like when?"

He replied, "April 5,2000. It will cost you $868.00"

My heart jumped, I took a deep breath and asked,

"For real, are you sure?"

He answered, "Yes sir, would you like for me to confirm that?"

I said," Yes. When and where do I pay the money?"

He said, "You have 24 hours to pay the money,
Either through a credit card, or Western Union." I told him,
"I prefer western union!"

He went over some general information with me and we hung up.

I praised Jehovah for his blessing and oversight over the matter.

I called Sonita and told her the deal.

She sounded much better over the phone; especially once she knew I was really paying for them to get back.

Sonita said, "You really love me, don't you?" I told her,
"Of course, you are my world." She then asked me,
"Are you gonna change once I get back?" I asked her,
"For what? My only change will be a good one." She said,
"Yeah, right Bay. I can't wait to feel your dick all up in me.

I miss how you suck and pump my pussy." I excitedly told her,
"Stop it, just stop it. You got me getting harder than a truck load of frozen neck bones! Customers are here, Sonita. Please stop playing with my mind."

She just burst out laughing real hard to the point where I ended up laughing with her.

I hung up with her and finished cutting. I made $100.00 today.

Thursday morning I paid $880.00 to bring my family back to me. Thursday night I made $100.00. Friday I made $125.00. Saturday I made $185.00 I paid my rent man $300.00 and said, "you'll have the rest next week."

Monday I paid my $75.00 booth rent.

Right then, I got on my knees and thanked Jehovah for helping me through. I couldn't have done it without him.

I am an eye witness that Jehovah is <u>real</u>, as many times I have placed my trust in him, he has <u>**NEVER**</u> failed me yet.

I put together the coming home party for Sonita. It was scheduled to go down at Crescent Apartments, through this janitorial dude whose hair I cut. However, the closer it came to the time the more he was fronting on the confirmation of the date.

I'm calling her in the meantime and she keeps going back and forth with me. Basically through the week she was coming home and our conversation is peace. Once the weekend comes she doesn't want to come back. Right then I knew, Oh dude was still hitting that. I was hoping she wouldn't get spoiled by the dick and catch the fuck its. Sexually, I couldn't please her, she was too far away. However, spiritually, mentally, and emotionally I could. I did the best I could until April came around.

I was very nervous because I didn't know whether she was really going to be on that flight.

That other guy was digging her and she was feeling him.

I got in contact with Jazz. I needed a big truck to bring her stuff back in; only if she is on this plane. April sixth was the arrival date. She left April fifth. I get up first thing in the morning. I call Jazz he's on his way. I'm as sharp as I can possibly be. We leave and get to the airport. We go to the place where she is supposed to land.

I give Jazz my camcorder so he can film my historical day.

The big question, is she on this flight, or not?

The passengers started coming off the plane although I don't see my peoples.

I turn around to Jazz and he's fumbling with the recorder.

I help him fix the vision, then I walk back over to see if any more people are getting off the plane. When they came through the door my heart jumped like the first time I laid eyes on her.

My sons looked so handsome and bright.

I thanked Jehovah constantly for bringing her back.

I knew then she was gonna be my wife. We hugged and kissed for the first time in eight months. I grabbed for my sons. I couldn't resist from picking Abijah up. He had my baby smile.

He was big and handsome. I told Jazz, "Make sure you get this fella." I reached for Jehdiah but, he just stayed under his mother.

Jazz said, "He a little shy he will come around."

Sonita said, "Jehdiah was the main one talking to you on the phone, now check him out."

I just kept staring at Abijah, he was so big. I told Jazz, "Get a close up of him. In the meantime, Jehdiah kept staring at me.

Jazz said, "Lets go down stairs to get her things, by the way we didn't get no tongue action on the camera." We all laughed.

Then we got her things and loaded them in Jazz truck, and finally rolled out.

Then it registered to Jehdiah by the time we got home that, I was his Daddy. Sonita was so shocked to see how Abijah just took to me.

She said, "Love, don't you know that Abijah would fight or cry if someone tried to pick him up. It's amazing how he senses that you are his daddy.

He didn't cry or anything. He just laid on you."

We chilled at the house, and Sonita surprised me with a gift.

She bought me clothes, cologne, and a souvenir.

I propose to her again in my kitchen, and she said, "Yes." then I took my sons and her to my job.

I cut Abijah's hair. He didn't cry or move. He was as still as a grown up. I knew he was my blood because all of my sons were like that. Sonita met Alicia, who I called "Jersey" because we were from the same hometown. It was peace. Alicia was telling Sonita how much I was in love with her. I never stopped talking about her.

She joked me about when I didn't think Sonita was coming back.

I was looking sick. They laughed together but I was embarrassed.

Sonita was happy and content with her family, not to mention the fact that we now shared a beautiful thing.

We attended our meetings, we went to the movies every other weekend. We took our sons to the parks, the malls, and the beach together. People would see us out in public and walk right up to us and say, "You look so happy together, your children are so nice and manageable; how do you keep control over them so well?"

We would blush and give the praise to Jehovah. Others would be shocked about our ages. Some thought we were high school kids with our little brothers or nephews. She would explain,

"He's my fiancé; he's 30 and I'm 22. We've been together since 1994."

My divorce became final April 13, 2000. My lawyer called me after his vacation on April 24th. He said,

"Mr Barkley this is Ronald Zed, you can come to my office and pick up your divorce papers." I asked,

"I could?" and his reply was simply,

"Yes."

Sonita and I went to pay our bills and pick up the papers.

We planned our day on April 25, 2000 and we carried it out. We spoke to one another meaning our vows from the bottom of our hearts.

Jehdiah and Abijah were there, and we had a ball!

We went to Apple Bees, ate, and then came home. We put our boys to bed and made love the whole night through.

From then on, we were looking for a bigger place.

Sonita secured her a job at Seven Eleven out in Ocean View. There she ran into her Uncle, on her father's side, and he told her where her father was.

She wanted me to go around there with her. I did, they met and kicked it but Sonita still didn't feel any better about him.

She could see right through his excuses and that made her dislike him more.

She felt he could've just admitted his wrong and done better; after all, she was grown now.

Nonetheless he didn't step up at all.

May came around and we were shining. I planned to take her to the Bobbie Womack Concert for Mother's Day. It was a surprise by then. I had a welcome home party for her at the barbershop. She saw from all of my customers that I was about her. She felt good. The box she mailed to me from Hawaii came on a boat to my house.

When we went through it, there were pictures of the guy she had slept with, plus another guy who she went out with.

I was hurt and disappointed. It seemed like all I was doing for her didn't matter. Once she saw how crushed I was,

Sonita apologized for even keeping and sending the pictures to my home. Then, she told me, "Look Love, I lied to you.

I called Patrick sense I been home. He thinks we are getting back together once they station him in V.A.

I lead you and him on.

I didn't know if we were gonna make it, so I kept him as a back up plan. I'm sorry Bay."

I was speechless. Tears were just pouring down my cheeks while she spoke.

I asked, "Do you want to be with him now? Sobbing.

She said, "No, I married you. You are the man I want."

I told her,

"Well, tell him. It's no need for you to play with his feelings.

He deserves to know the truth." She nonchalantly said,

"I ain't got to tell him, he'll get over it." I said to her,

"Sonita that's not right. Plus I can't get over it.

Call him and put my mind at ease. Let him know you are married."

She was scared to death. It took her two hours before she would call the dude.

I couldn't believe I was going through this.

In the mist of us waiting for her to call, her brother Eric rode past. She yelled out his name and he doubled back.

We talked for a minute. He informed her that he was down the block at his girl's spot. He was very busy; practically working two jobs.

He assured her, though, that he would come by to see her.

After that, he left and she called ol' dude.

She told him what time it was and then hung up. She cried afterwards and said, "I don't ever want to go through that again."

I said, "Me either. I have some tickets to the Bobby Womack concert. I want to take you there for Mothers Day."

She just started crying more." After the tears subsided she asked me, "Love, why do you put up with me?" I told her,

"Sonita, it's obvious I love you. I've done wrong things in my life and you stuck it out with me. I know for a fact that there's no other woman who love's me like you do."

I took her to the show and we had a ball, we were shining!

When we got home, I pulled out my money I had saved from cutting. It was close to $9,000.00 and Sonita was shocked.

She through the money in the air. Then, she wanted me to take pictures of her and the money. We had fun. This was the life I always dreamed I would have with my soul mate. We were in love and it felt great!

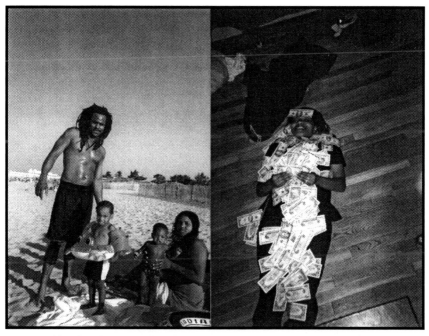

ERIC LONEY, JEHDIAH, ABIJAH, AND SONITA, at Ocean view Beach. June, 2000

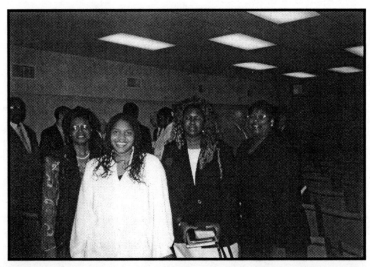
Sonita at the kingdom hall, after she came back from Hawaii.

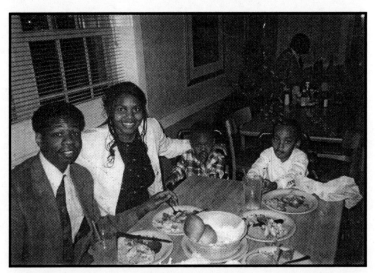
RANDELL, SONITA, ABIJAH, AND JEHDIAH,
eating dinner at Golden Carol after coming from the Kingdom Hall.

June comes around and Sonita is still working at Seven Eleven.

We kept going to the Kingdom Hall. Bro and Sister Capo were studying with us the Family Book. Sonita would go out to the beach and visit her family on the weekends. Things were cool.

July came and we took our sons to Water Country. Sometimes we would get her twin cousins and they would have fun with us.

In the meantime, I'm still in the shop working.

However, at times, Sonita would pop up at my job thinking she would catch me cheating on her. For no apparent reason, she couldn't believe that I was faithful to her. That used to hurt me to my heart because everything I did wrong in my first marriage, I did better this time around. Some women would stop by just to speak. But Sonita would diss them and say "If you're not getting a service, I don't want you talking to my husband." I told Sonita, "You can't do that because you will ruin business for me. I deal with the public on a day- to- day basis and it's not always a service people get. Some people just want to talk. And get things off their chest. Sonita didn't care so 40% of my woman customers I lost. It bothered me, however I knew I didn't do nothing wrong.

I figured eventually she will see. Then it dawn on me, maybe it's her conscience eating a way at her. She is being very controlling over me. Jehdiah and Abijah love coming to the shop and play.

One day Sonita left around 7 to start dinner. I told her" I'd be home by 9. It started raining real hard so around 8:30 I started shutting the shop down. Nasseem came running in the shop to get out of the rain. He was a young kid around 15. He told me.

"Love can I stay in here for a while, my parent's aint home and I can't get in." I said,

"Well, you can chill for a minute, my wife just made dinner and I have to go home." He asked,

"Can I go home with you? At least until my moms get home?" I said, "First I have to ask wifee, I got to go past Block Busters to pick up a movie for us to watch. Now, while I'm there you can call your moms and see if she's home. If she's not then I'll take you with me, and when she does get there, I'll just run you back okay?"

He said, "Okay."

I called Sonita and told her what was going on. She didn't have a problem with it. However, she informed me it's only enough food for us. I told her, "That's cool, he just wants to get out of the rain." We went to Block Busters on Hampton Blvd.

I got the movies she wanted. Then we called to his house from a pay phone. His mother was home so I ran him home and drove myself home. I got there around 10pm Sonita is mad.

"So, where is Nasseem?" She asked. I told her,

"I dropped him off once we left Block Busters.

His parents were home." She screamed,

"You know you are a lying ass mother fucker! I know you was with a bitch!" I innocently exclaimed,

"No I wasn't! I told you Nasseem was with me. You can call his house and ask his moms if I didn't just drop him off." Then she yelled, "That's bullshit, he will probably lie for you!"

I curiously asked, "Sonita what is your problem; I asked you before I left the shop.

I was going to take him with me , you were cool with it." Then she asked, "Well, where is he?" I exclaimed again,

"His parents came home!"

She didn't believe me so she took the dinner she had cooked and threw the whole pot of food out the window.

I shouted at her, "Why did you do that?"

With a very nasty attitude she said,

"Get that bitch you was with to make you something."

My sons started crying and I went to comfort them.

Sonita pushed me away from them. Then she punched me dead in the face. I grabbed. her hands and we started wrestling to the floor.

Our sons are screaming now. I tell her, "Look cut this shit out in front of the kids." She said,

"No, motherfucker." She hit me in my nuts. I picked her up and threw her on our bed. I tried to pin her down, but she kept fighting harder and harder. We fell off the bed and she hit her head. She started screaming "You made me hit my head, I hate you!" I asked,

"Sonita what is wrong with you?"

She got off the floor and ran into the kitchen to get a knife.

Quickly I jumped out the window.

I went and called Bro Johnson.

I told him what was going on, he told me," Take it up with God and try to work it out."

I said, "This girl is crazy for real. She has change since she came from to Hawaii, I don't know her any more."

Bro Johnson patiently said,

"Randell, you have to exercise patience with her; you're older and more mature."

I saw he wasn't understanding me so I hung up with him.

I went back to the house and she wouldn't let me in.

Confused, I left and got a room out in Ocenview.

I called her and tried to talk to her, but she didn't want to talk.

The next day I went back to the house. The window was open so I climbed through it. She was on the phone talking with her sister. Sonita told her she will talk to her later. The boys ran straight to me. I hugged them, then I walked over to her. I asked her, "Why did you fight me Sonita? I didn't do any thing wrong.

I love you. I wasn't with any girl." She asked,

"Whatever Love; you didn't have to make me hit my head." I told her, "That was an accident and you know it." She said,

"I'm tired of fighting with you Love, I just remember how we met and got together. I'm thinking you'll probably be with some one else." I said to her,

"Sonita, I don't want no body but you! Can't you see that?

No girl has ever approach you over me, you don't find numbers in my pockets, and you know everywhere I go. I don't leave you in the dark, but you will take my sons and I don't see you for two days!!?

I don't jump to conclusions thinking you are with a dude.

You tell me you're with your family, and I believe you.

I tell you Nasseem needed my help, and I'm lying."
She sadly said,
"I don't know Love I do overreact sometimes, but I know it's woman out there who want you." I told her,
"And, what am I, that naive to just give myself to anyone who likes me. Like I can't say no. Come on Sonita, we been together too long for that. I'm sorry for fighting with you but, you start it every time." Out of no where the phone rang, it was her sister calling back. I told her we were talking and she will holla at her later. She asked me,
"Love, do you want to watch the movie you got last night?"
I said, "Yes Sonita."
We laid up in the bed with our sons and threw in the movie.
Thirty minutes later it's a knock at the door.
I look out the window and it's the police.
I said, "What the fuck? You called the cops on me? And you're the one who caused the confrontation."
She jumped up to go downstairs to open the door.
I followed her.
Sonita started yelling at me, "You shouldn't a hit me." I said,
"Dead it Sonita, we were just in here watching a movie, now you're flipping."
I opened the door and they asked me my name and I told them.
They then told me I was under arrest for assault.
I said "This is some bull shit! I haven't assaulted her.
Dig, before you take me, let me get my jacket it's on the door.
Sonita was already standing by my jacket. The police told her to hand me my jacket. She did. I said, "Hold up officer, my wallet and keys are missing. Inside my wallet is a $100 dollar bill and two $50 dollar bills." They ask her, "Do you have his wallet and keys?" She said,
"Yes here it is." She handed my keys and wallet to the officer although my money was gone.
I told them, "Hold up, check her, she got my money."

The male officer questioned her and she denied having my money. So they took me to jail. I was hurt to my heart. I thought to myself she is cheating on me. She's probably still talking to that dude in Hawaii.

The Magistrate let me go on my own recognizance and told me I couldn't go to the house for 72 hours.

I called Samad and told him what happened. He paid for a cab to bring me to his house. He loaned me some money in order for me to get a room for the next couple of days.

I knew I had to go back to my place because I had three grand stashed in the house. If she would take my last, I know she will take all my cash.

When she went to work, I went to the apartment. My two vcrs, cam recorder, key boards, lap top, T.V. and car were gone.

The house was a wreck, but she didn't find my money.

To her knowledge I was still locked up.

I went to work and started cutting. My client name Trannie came in. I told him what happened, and he said his wife, he had just married, was taking him through the same thing.

We were both bugging' because we used to talk about our girls to each other. His girl was in Florida and Sonita was in Hawaii.

We used to call them like crazy. Now, we get them to us and they start wilding. After that, he left and went home. One hour later, he calls me and say,

"Love, your car is in front of my building." I asked him,

"Are you sure it's my car?" He said,

"Yes. Love I'll come through and scoop you."

We went to his building and my car was there with all my shit in it. I took my car to my job and twenty minutes later Sonita called me from work saying," I know you got the car." I asked her,

"How do you know that? Who are you fucking with out there?"

She said," Nobody." I said,

"Your lying, you got somebody watching my car. If I find out you're fucking around Sonita, I'm a fuck you up for real and I'm a turn my self in.

I don't deserve this treatment from you. All I ever did was love you." She replied,

"Well, I want to move." I said,

"I bet you do, now that you know I'm for real."

That night she came to my apartment, she told me,

"I'm staying with my cousin out in the beach. Some Spanish people I met babysat our sons while I was at work.

The girl lives in the building where your car was."

I asked her," So you were going to sell my shit, for what? We are a family, so where is all this bullshit coming from. Tell me who are you fucking with?"

She said," Nobody." I said,

"Okay when we go to court for this situation you better tell them the truth. You started it."

She sheepishly said, "I will Love."

The next month we went to court and she told the truth. However, the prosecutor said, "Sonita is probably scared of Mr. Barkley and that's why she changed her statement."

Sonita told them, "I'm not scared of my husband, I love him and need him free to take care of us. It's really my fault."

So the prosecutor asked for a recess. She talked to us outside. She was trying to convince me to take the charge and I'll get probation. I said, "Hell no. My wife told you the truth, what more do you want?" The prosecutor said to us,

"Well the judge takes cases like this serious. I will tell him you plead no contest; which means he can find you guilty and your pay a fine and be order to attend anger management classes."

I protested, "That's not fair, I didn't do nothing."

Sonita said, "Can I attend anger management classes instead of him?" The prosecutor asked,

"Why Mrs. Barkley, that would be double the money your husband will have to pay." For that reason, I said,

"Okay, I'll say no contest, let's get this over with."

I was ordered to pay $360.00 and do 18 weeks in anger management classes.

Sonita felt terrible for doing this to me. I had it made up in my mind, once I finished this shit I'm out; due to the fact that Sonita is draining me, and I can't take it no more.

She started a new job out in Chesapeake doing customer service.

Things started going smoother, now that she had a better job and less time to harass me at work.

We started going back to the meetings.

Then she wrote me another letter it read………………………………

The letter made my day because I really felt like I was a sucker to be in this relationship. I didn't think she appreciated me .

I started my classes and we began our plan to move.

We needed a bigger place for the boys and I needed space for my equipment. We saved up our money and in June 2001 we found a loft, condo apartment in Norfolk.

We were so happy when they approved us to move in.

Our first night there was so beautiful. We watched Jehdiah and Abijah chase each other all through the house. They were jumping up and down, laughing and singing. I started chasing Sonita around and our sons were laughing at us, afterwards we cooked a big dinner for our family. We ate, then watched a Block Buster movie together. Finally, we put our sons to sleep and made love like it was our first time.

That night Shereef was conceived. We were vibrant as we could have ever been.

We had great times. We use to sit out side and just stare at the stars. Reminiscing about how we met. Sonita said,

"Remember Love when we walked on the rocks out on the beach in Ocean view?"

I paused and said, "Yes." She continued, "and we went inside the opening and there were fishes swimming in the lower water. Then we started kissing." I smiled and said, "That was a crazy day, and as soon as we started doing the nasty, a big rat ran by us and we jetted out of there!"

We both began to laugh. Sonita said, "Them were fun times, you use to rap and sing to me." Then I hugged her from behind and we stared into space. I started singing R Kelly song to her, *"sit down on the couch, take your shoes off, let me rub your body before I tear it off the homey lover man is ready to flex girl flex time to have sex.*

We laughed and she turn around to face me and said, "I love you. I said, "I love you too." Afterwards we went in the house, made love, then went to sleep. We both had to get up in the morning.

We both were working. Sonita met our next door neighbor. She was a nice woman with two sons. They got along good with our sons. We all became friends.

We were making our meetings. Jehdiah and Abijah loved the Kingdom Hall. They loved the witnesses.

We felt their genuine love for us.

The sisters from Hawaii used to write her, as well as send pictures.

I bought another car. We had three cars to commute with.

Sonita invited her family that stays in Virginia Beach over to see her. However , Billy, who lives in Maryland, was the first family member to visit. The rest of the family didn't see him.

Sometimes he'd just come to see us and we got along good.

Billy reminded me a lot of my brother Ibn; a people person.

Eventually, her aunts and cousin came around. They enjoyed them selves here. Jehdiah was always under Aunt Annette.

Abijah would stay to himself. When other kids were around Abijah, he would boo guard.

I started getting my studio equipment in place. Spoon inspired me to do that. We recorded, "Hard Times" and "757;" and it was on.

All of my friends and family were coming through this summer.

Vernon, Cutter, Mohammed, Ibn, Dog, Droop, Treyindoe, Jazz, Samad, Naseem, and a couple of others.

I made dinner early so I could work on this song about Sonita.

I had the big kool aid smile all day long just by thinking of her. I went upstairs into my lab and I came up with this song called "Homey Loving Friend." I got the concept from R Kelly's song.

It took me back to the times when we first met. It was about Sonita and how good our relationship is.

While I was working on the song, Jehdiah was downstairs laughing his tail off to the road runner show.

He had me weak with laughter. I wrote the first verse..

> *There's nothing better than having someone special,*
> *without strings attached, you are my chosen vessel.*
> *you been down for the ride, and by my side*
> *Remember wifie came home early ,and you had to hide.*
> *Damn girl, I know you really must love me*
> *to stay in the closet that long, putting up with the heat.*
> *But don't get me wrong cause my love is strong,*
> *You have me mesmerized how your body bounce in that thong.*
> *I like it rough and sweaty you like it hard and steady*
> *doggy style the way you shout have me going crazy,*
> *but sometimes you can get out of place*
> *I just spoke to the chick, you didn't have to smash her face.*
> *you know out side of wifie you're, the only one*
> *who get my time and my money, baby girl, you're fun.*
> *you accept my life, my wife, and my children,*
> *so what more can I ask for in a homey loving friend.*

Then Sonita came home from work. Jehdiah ran to her as usual.

Abijah always tried to hang but never could make it, so Jehdiah really eats up all the attention he can get. She spoke,

"Hey Bay, what are you doing?" I said,

"Working on a song." In the meantime, she is coming up the stairs. Jehdiah is right with her. I'm still typing the song.

She looks over my shoulder to read it.

She said, "Who is this girl you are talking about?"

I said," You, Sonita damn!"

She replied, "No it's not, I never stayed up in no closet!"

I said, "I was just being funny Sonita.

But everything else is you." I grinned.

She said, "Yeah right, you be exaggerating hah, hah!"

I continued, "It's all a part of telling the story. What, you don't like it?" She said,

"No! I didn't say that, it's nice Bay I see where you're going with it." I said,

"Thanks." We hugged and kissed. Then I said,

"Sonita your dinner is in the stove."

She said, "That's good Bay, you cooked dinner?"

I said,"Yeah, I know I was gonna order out, but I decided to cook."

She asked, "You read my letter?"

I said, "Yes Sonita, it was nice and I'd like to cash in."

She chuckled and smiled, then went downstairs with Jehdiah.

She and Jehdiah ate while she informed me about her day at work. Jehdiah fell asleep and we made love.

The following day, I get a call from my cousin Ronnie.

He says, "Yo cuz, I'm on my way down there! What's up, its me and Stan you heard.

We got a room down at the beach and we're trying to party!

Call Jazz and let him know its on!" I said,

"Word cuz I'm with it. I know you gonna come to my house first?

See the family and the new spot. You know."

Sonita asked me, "Who is that?"

I said,"Ronnie, he's coming down with one of his friends."

She said, "Word, tell him I said Hi"

I said to him, "Ronnie Wifie said hi."

He then said," Give her my love." I said to her,

"He sends his love. Look Sonita he wants me to go out with them. I'm a ride with him to Jazz house okay?" She said,

"That's cool Love, you know you gonna have to be back before I go to work." I said,

"I know. Rah, how long before ya'll get here?"

He said," About 2 hour's son, you heard?"

I said, "Bet." Then we hung up.

I called Jazz and told him he was hype.

Sonita walked into the kitchen and started cooking and I began to clean up. The boys were running around playing with their friends next door. Their moms came over and kicked it with Sonita.

Meanwhile, Jazz called me back saying he wanted us to go to this event with him. I told him I was with it, but I had my sons to watch. Two hours later Ronnie called me asking for directions to my spot.

I told him. They were in a white Lexus with some phat rims on them.

They came inside and ate dinner with us as Ronnie was informing me on the family. He had us all laughing at the top of our lungs!

I told Sonita, "I'll be back in three hours."

She said," Ronnie, you make sure he gets back in time for me to go to work." He said,

"You got that cuz, we gonna get Jazz and hang out for a minute. I'll have him back."

We left and went to Jazz's house. There we played basketball, and reminisced on our past.

Afterwards, we left to get back to my house. Jazz said he would meet up with us later. The radio station was bigging up a club out in the beach. Ronnie and Stan wanted to check it out. I told them I had to take my sons with me ,so I won't be able to go in the club, but I could hang out with ya'll on the strip.

We made it back in three hours. Sonita was almost ready to leave.

I pulled out the playing cards and we played three hand spades.

Sonita asked me, "Are they spending the night?" I replied,

"No, they got rooms down at the beach." She said,

"Oh well I'm a see ya'll fellas when I get off from work."

The children and I gave her a hug and kiss afterwards she bounced.

I played music and enjoyed my family's company.

Ronnie spoke, "Yo cuz, come with us out to the beach so we can change for tonight. That way, once we chill with you on the strip, we can shoot you and your son's home. Then, we are gonna do our thing. You heard?"

"That's what's up Rah, we can leave after the game."

We hit the highway and coasted down to the beach.

It was packed everywhere. On our way, I'm in the back seat with my son's free styling. We were having a ball.

Once we hit the strip we had to drive slow. Meanwhile, cars are passing us and girls are hollering. Out of the blue some girls in the next car flashed their tities at us. Stan came to a stop and yelled at the girls to pull over.

They said, "turn around!"

Stan scream back, "alright!"

As a result bike cop rides up on us and tells Stan to pull over.

He asked, "For what?"

The cop said, "You are blocking traffic."

Stan blurted out," No I'm not, traffic aint even moving."

Two more bike cops come over and asked,

"What seems to be the problem?"

They replied," This guy is blocking traffic."

Stan said, "I told your ass I'm not blocking shit, and I haven't broken any laws."

Another cop looked in the back of the car and said, "Whose beer is that?"

I said, "It's mine officer."

His next replied was, "Are these your children too?"

I said, "Yes."

Rah and Stan were flipping on the cops hard. Rah kept his cam recorder running the whole time.

My phone rang! It was Sonita. One cop told me to get out of the car. I said, "For what?"

He said,"Im going to search the car for weapons."

Stan responded with, "No your not. You can run my info, but your not searching my whip for shit!"

I answered the phone. "Hi Sonita are you on your break?"

She said, "Yes Bay, I want to talk to you."

I said to her, "Well, Sonita I really can't talk right now, but on your next break I'll rap with you." She raised her voice and said,

"What you mean you can't talk, I know you ain't with no bitch!"

I screamed out," Hell no!! I'll explain it to you later o.k.?"

She continued, "No Love, tell me what's going on, I hate it when you get brand new around your cousin!"

I said, "Here we go with this shit, that's not true."

The cop told me, "Sir get off the phone now, we are conducting an investigation."

Sonita couldn't hear him, however she can hear the crowd in the background. People all loud walking pass.

She said, "You got some bitches at my house!"

I said, "No Sonita stop bugging the fuck out."

Then the cop told me, "Cut it short." So I hung up.

In the meantime, Rah and Stan are still going off on the other cops for harassing us.

After having us pulled over for an hour, they let us go.

That basically killed the hour or two I wanted to spend with my family.

We went to their room and they changed. Afterwards we left, and rode back to Norfolk.

Once we get there Rah said," Love aint that Sonita?"

I said, "Where?"

He pointed and said, "Look, on the balcony."

With confusion and shock I said, "Yeah, that's her, she's supposed to be at work. I know this girl didn't leave work just to check up on me?"

We parked and went up stairs. She's mad.

She started screaming, "Where have you been?"

I cut her off and said, "Fuck where I've been, why you aren't at work?"

She sarcastically said," See how you act around you family?"

I said, "Sonita,whatever bullshit you on, you really need to dead it."

As we walk in the house, she is cursing me out and making a scene.

I pull her in our room and tell her, "Long as we been together you still got doubts about my loyalty to you? You wild out on my family, left your job and came all the way home, for what?

Are any girls here, no! Matter a fact, I don't want to talk about it.

Yo Rah, show her the tape."

Sonita looked puzzled and said," What tape Love?"

I continued, "Hold on Sonita, Rah go ahead and show her."

He rewinded the video tape and played it for her.

She saw with her own eyes what happened, plus she was able to hear when my phone rang and my conversation with her, while the cops surrounded us.

She felt real stupid and childish to have left work on an assumption.

I told her, "You might as well go back to work."

She refused. She just apologized for her actions and went to sleep. Rah said, "Well she's home now, you think she'll let you roll?"

I said, "Shit, not in this lifetime."

Stan and Rah just laughed and left.

The one night with my cousin was ruined.

I just took it down and went to sleep.

The next day she still didn't go to work.

I told her, "Sonita, I need you to work so we can manage our spot."

She said, "I know Bay, but I really don't like that job."

I reasoned with her and said, "I understand that, but get another job before you quit."

She softly replied, "I'll get a job don't worry." Then she started feeling on my dick. I gently pushed her hand away and said,

"I got to worry, because you are putting more pressure on me; all you have to do is go back to work."

She didn't do it. Two months went by and we find out she's pregnant again. In the meantime her friends from the job started coming by from time to time. The guy who own's the shop I work at was arrested. I ended up going to Pat's Barbershop to work. That was a big adjustment for me because, I was first, used to being in a shop alone.

Second, I work on Mondays and they didn't, therefore the $100.00 I made that day was gone. Third, my rent was higher and the shop was smaller. Four, half of my clients didn't like one of the barbers who worked there so they wouldn't come to the shop.

Some were willing to come to my home than to come in the shop. However, I don't cut out of my home so I lost them.

Five, was weekly I grossed $750.00 but now it's down to $400 a week. I was primarily starting from scratch, with the support of 50% of my clientele. Pat was a good boss though, he let me live my first week there.

I got along great with everyone who worked there and that was peace also. It was Pat, Mink, Jessica, who they called Jay and myself. They met my family and everything was cool. Then after about two weeks of working there Sonita was mad.

She said," Why you always came home late?"

I responded with," I have to stay late to catch the late comers nobody want to cut. I'm trying to build my clientele back up, plus you're not working.

I have to make up for your income that I need to pay our bills."

She said, "Yeah right, I know you probably fucking that girl who works there."

I said, "Come on Sonita don't start that stuff up again."

She said, "I see how she looks at you, do she be there late too?"

I said, "Sonita everybody be there, It isn't just us two."

She said, "Yeah right love, I can't take it no more get the fuck out!"

I sadly said," You are bugging Sonita; every time you get pregnant you start this shit. No I'm not leaving; I'm hungry and I want to eat."

She said," You talk to her though? right! Right!"

I said,"Sonita, I talk to everybody, not just her."

She screamed out," I knew it I knew it! It's more bitches huh?"

I yelled back," Hell no! Everybody in the shop damn!"

She screamed back, "Get out now, before I call the police!"

My heart dropped and the first thing popped in my head was what the director of the anger management class said, "If your girl start acting irate and threatens you, just leave. <u>Walk away.</u>"

I said, "Fine, Sonita, I'll go." My sons started crying,

"Don't go daddy stay, come on stay."

I said, "Sorry fellas, I'll be back."

She said, "You better not come back!"

I left, got in my car and drove away. I didn't have any where to go. I really didn't want any one in my business therefore I rode to Hampton boulevard and 35street. I pulled into the parking lot across from the cab company and went to sleep in my car.

The next morning, I went to get some breakfast from Donut Dinette on 20street and Colley avenue. Afterwards I went to work, cranky and adjitated, but no one could tell. Around 3 'O'clock in the afternoon, Sonita showed up at my job. She said, "Love come out side I need to talk to you."

I said," O.k."

My client name Bryant said, "She looks mad, what's up?"

I said, "Nothing I'll be right back."

I go out side and walks to the car where I could see Jehdiah and Abijah in the backseat jumping up and down.

They are very happy to see me.

Sonita spoke, "Where have you been?"

I said, "What, didn't you put me out? It shouldn't matter to you where I've been."

She spoke more aggresive,"Love I'm serious, I want to know, you didn't come back at all last night."

I said to her, "For what, so we could argue and you can lie like you did before and have me locked up? Sonita, I don't have time for this shit! I got five more weeks of this program left and I'm not gonna let you jam me up."

She pouted,"Fuck that Love, where did you sleep?"

I replied, "In my car where else?"

Then she said," You was with that bitch at your job wasn't you?

That's why you didn't come back home!"

I told her, "I don't even know her, or where she lives, so stop it.

You are going to come to my job with all this drama and I just started working here?"

She screamed out, "Love tell me the truth; matter a fact, I'm a ask her."

I said, "Sonita don't you dare embarrass me after how highly I talked about us to everyone."

She continued, "You been talking about me to her?"

I screamed out, "No, Sonita to the guys o.k."

She said, "I don't believe you" Then she walked passed me and went in the shop and called Jay outside.

She asked her, "Jay are you fucking my husband?"

Jay quickly replied, "No! I don't even know Love like that."

Sonita then said, "Did he stay at your house last night, and don't fucking lie to me!"

Jay continued," No, no, no, we work together and he left before me. Sonita I have a man I don't want yours." Then Jay turned around and walked back in the shop.

I sadly said,"Sonita I can't believe you ask her that! Why are you causing a scene at my job? Are you trying to get me fired?"

She said, "Love you was some where with a bitch and when I find her I'm a kill her!"

I told her," You are tripping for real" Then she grabbed me by the neck and scratch blood out of me and ripped my shirt off my back in front of the barbershop and our children. I didn't even put up a fight. I just walked away. She followed behind me and punched me in the back.

I grabbed her and held her close that way she couldn't hurt me any more.

I yelled out, "Stop it please, Sonita you done embarrass me enough."

Then she started crying screaming, "You wont tell me where you been you must've been with a girl!"

I told her,"Sonita no I wasn't I slept in the car on Hampton boulevard and 35street that way I could go to work and don't be late."

She softly said," For real, why didn't you just say that?"

I said," First of all, you are the one who put me out. Now you want to be concerned about where I been?"

She said, "I didn't mean it Love, but I don't see you that much."

I said, "Sonita you're the reason, you left your job, I can't be home early and pay bills. You need to go to anger management class for real.

You jump to conclusions and convince yourself it's the truth without proof.

If I wanted somebody else I wouldn't a married you.

All this bragging I was doing about our great marriage done went out the window. For what? If you just keep yourself busy and tend to the boys we will be alright."

In the meantime Bryant got in Pats chair so he could finish his cut.

I popped my trunk therefore I could put on another shirt. Sonita apologizes for her action and promise not to overreact again.

I told her, "If you put me out, or call the police on me again, <u>I will leave you for real</u>, I can't live like this. You're draining me baby.

Its like I'm a boxer, and my opponent is the job world, and you are my trainer. After each round the boxer goes to his corner for advice, water and rest for that minute. Then, after being refreshed he fights another round. But how could I win if when I return to my corner you give me discouragement, fire and no chair for me to rest. I will easily be defeated. Sonita, that's what you're doing to me.

I come home for love, nourishment, and affection. That way I can be equipped to work another day. We are partners, lovers, parents, and friends. I don't want that to end. But, if you continue to push me away there's nothing I can do but leave."

While we are talking, Pat comes out and say, "Is everything alright?"

Sonita spoke, "Yes everything is cool I'm leaving soon."

Then she smiled and said,

"Love ,I don't know what came over me, it's like now that I'm pregnant again I see things different. I don't think you want me any more. You spend more time with our sons than you do with me.

Or your working on building your studio. When am I gonna get some attention? I'm sorry for wilding at your job, look Bay, I'll talk to you tonight alright? Are you coming home?"

I calmly said, "Yes Sonita, I am, but first let me hugg and kiss my boys."

She sadly said, "Well, what about me? Can I get a hugg and kiss too?"

I smiled and said, "Of course." We hugged and kissed then she left.

I went back in the shop and they all asked me why she was bugging out. They saw the blood coming from my neck and chest. I just walk in the bathroom and freshing up. When I came out I said "She pregnant that's why she's tripping. Everybody had their little comments to say, however I really didn't pay it no mind.

I was depress for the whole day. I turned down three heads and went home early. We talked about it more when I got home.

Sonita made me dinner, and we watched a movie together.

Then we went to sleep.

The next day she started looking for a part-time job and I went to work. The next couple of weeks went fine.

I got my studio in effect and I started recording my album.

Spoon and I were hanging out more. We were learning the equipment together. Vernon was coming through giving us pointers. He gave me a job assembling furniture.

That was a big help on my bills.

Muhammad was moving up top so he sold me his furniture for cheap.

Our place was nice and peaceful now. However, it was hard for me to know how her mood might be once I got home.

I was in love with her so it didn't matter to me. I rather deal with her than any body else because overall Sonita was a great person. She loved her sons and me. We were her world and she didn't want no one coming in between it. Our family and friends stopped coming around like they used to. Basically to give us our space. Her back started hurting her and she started feeling depressed. Then her child hood would haunt her and make her feel down.

She felt sad that her cousins her age had their parents, and everything they wanted. However, she didn't. Her grandfather died, he was her mother and father put together.

She felt very lonely inside.

This was one reason why she was so over protective of me.

She didn't want no one taking me away from her, because I was everything to her. That's why she wanted a child so bad, so she could have someone to love that was hers, and she knew would love her back. We seemed to talk about these things every time she gets pregnant. I listen, comfort her and let her cry her heart out.

Then the next morning, we saw on the news about a lady in Texas who killed her children and tried to kill herself, but survived. The media portrayed her as crazy and the husband, as the cause, for her flipping. However, after her arrest the husband stood by her. I told Sonita, "She was crazy to do such a thing."

Sonita said, "Not really. I feel her. I be having thoughts about hurting our kids and killing myself." I said,

"Sonita you are bugging out now, life aint that bad to make you want to do such a thing." She continued,

"No Love, for real. I feel that way sometimes, but it goes away.

I just don't like how I was raised and why I have to suffer without, while everyone my age I know got. It really hurts sometimes."

I said, "Oh baby, don't feel like that, we love you, just wait until I get this record deal. I'm a buy you the world!"

After our conversation I left and went to work.

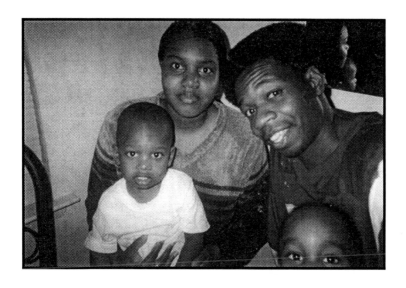

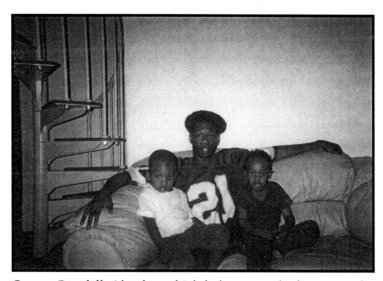

Sonita, Randell, Abijah, and Jehdiah at our 3 bedroom condo.

ELEVEN
Fourth Child

I GET A CALL from my Uncle Randy in New Jersey and he informs me that Jerrica will be placed into the system if no one in the family takes her. I agreed to get her. That was plan for the next month. Sonita didn't have a problem with it, actually she was feeling Jerrica's pain because they were alike in many ways.

Both of them lost their parents at a young age and were going from house to house during her child hood.

The only difference was Jerrica has been molested and abused all her life, to the point where she ended up in special ed and on medication. She was only 12, but had the mind of a 6 year old; she wasn't in her right grade, either.

When I came home from work, we watched a movie with our kids then we went to sleep.

The following day she went to visit her cousin Me Me to see her baby. She came back happy and radiant. She visited with the neighbors and we played Casino. Sonita won. Then I went upstairs to my studio and worked on another song. My sons came upstairs and they wanted to get on the microphone so I recorded them rapping.

It was so funny because you can barely understand what they were saying and they were serious with it.

Afterwards, we went to sleep. I went to work the next day and grind as usual. I came home and dinner was ready for me and Sonita was cool, like we used to be. Before we knew it, next month came around and I was on my way to pick up my cousin.

I haven't seen her since 1997. I got to Irvington New Jersey and went pass my grandmother's house first, that way I could see my brothers.

After that, I went to pick Jerrica up. I talked to my uncle and his wife. They informed me of the crazy things that Jerrica did.

They even took me to the school to meet her teachers.

They basically told me I was in for a world of problems with her.

I felt she was probably so rebellious because she can sense no one was showing her genuine love and concern.

We left from there and went to their apartment to get her.

Once I saw her, she looked just like her mother. I spoke and she spoke back politely. I said, "She can't be all that bad Randy."

He said, "Shit don't let her innocent look fool you."

We put her bags into my car and Randy checked my oil and brake fluid for the ride. We hit the road and was on our way.

Jerrica talked me the whole way to V.A.

Once she got to my home, she was shocked about how big my place was. She met the family. She and Sonita hit it off cool.

I enrolled her into school and her new life began.

Sonita took Jerrica to her family's house out in the beach and they gave her some clothes. She loved it down here.

She got along good with our children and was very helpful around the house. She was on Ritalin to calm her down because she would get very hyper. Other than that, she was fine.

Then three weeks after being with us, Sonita calls me at work sounding sad.

She said, in a crying tone, "Love, I need you to come home."

I asked,, "Why, what's wrong?"

She said, "I don't want to talk about it over the phone, please, can you come home?"

I said, "Sonita, I'm cutting hair, plus I got three guys waiting, can it wait until I finish them?"

She said, "No Love, after that cut come home o.k.?"

I said, "Alright Sonita I'll be there." Then I hung up.

I told my three other clients that I had an emergency and I needed them to come back later or the next day. They were disappointed, but understanding.

When I got home Sonita was sitting at the table holding her head. Jehdiah and Abijah were on the couch looking sad. Jerrica was upstairs.

I asked her, "What's wrong?"

She explained, "Love, when I went to the phone booth downstairs to call my cousin, I left Jerrica and the boys in the house. When I came back in, I saw Jerrica push Jehdiah off of her, then she tried to pull her pants up real fast. Abijah's and Jehdiah's pants were down to their ankles. Jehdiah was crying saying, "Stop it. Stop it." Abijah started running towards me saying, "Jerrica touched me wee wee, Jerrica touched me wee wee." He was pointing at his wee wee. I was in shock and disgusted. I screamed at her and smacked her. Love, I don't want her in my house.

She molested my babies!"

I was in shock. I felt terrible, I didn't know what to do.

I questioned her about it and she admitted it. Therefore I whipped her butt.

Then, I talked with her afterwards. I explained to her how wrong it was to do that. However, she's been molested since she was small so she doesn't see anything wrong with it.

I just brought her down here and I know the only place left is the system. Sonita will never trust her around the kids again.

Sonita was crushed with hurt and pain. She was never in a situation like this and it bothered her. I couldn't blame her but I knew I couldn't get rid of my cousin. I was all she had left.

Therefore I took her to a shrink. I set her up with counseling and I tried to get the system to help me with her.

Meanwhile, when I left Jerrica had to leave with me. If she stayed home and Sonita had to use the bathroom she would have the boys in the bathroom with her. My home became divided.

Jerrica started doing the same thing she was doing up in New Jersey in school. Then I realized it was a part of her make up.

That brought on a lot of stress to Sonita.

If I came home late from work or we have an argument, Sonita would put me out. Then, she would wake up Jerrica and tell her she had to leave with me. Now, I got to sleep in the car with my cousin. If I had enough money I would get a hotel room and we could sleep there, then I would have to take her to school in the morning.

January came around and Sonita started getting bigger. Her back started to hurt her quite a bit, so I would massage it at night.

I went with her to most of her doctor's appointments.

They always told her to take it easy. The ladies there would compliment us on how well behaved our sons were. In the meantime, Jerrica is doing better in school.

Sonita had her baby shower and some of her family was there.

It was nice and Sonita had a good time. I had to work, so once I got a break I ran home to speak, eat, drop off the shop gift and say my peace. Jehdiah and Abijah were having a ball playing with their cousins. Jerrica enjoyed herself as well.

By then we knew how to deal with Jerrica. She couldn't be left around any children; other than that, Jerrica was alright. She had to be supervised just like a child. Sonita's family still showed her love.

Sonita's cousin Billy got his hair cut from me and I informed him on the inside scoop of what's been going on. He was the only person in her family I could talk to. He and Sonita were real tight, and I knew if he talked to Sonita, she would listen.

It was hell on me trying to keep my family in order under these crazy circumstances and I needed help.

He encouraged me to stick it out and he promised me he would holler at Sonita.

Sonita received numerous gifts at her baby shower and she was happy.

Nothing made me feel more better than to just see Sonita's pretty smile.

Jazz, Teresa, Samad, and Jan came over later that night and we partied some more.

We played spades and watched videos all night.

This was a very happy day for us, because our families came together to celebrate the arrival of our fourth child.

Sonita shed tears of joy once we were alone.

We stayed up the rest of the night looking through her gifts.

Afterwards, we went to sleep.

February came around and I was finishing up with anger management class. They make you stand up at the end of the term and comment on what you learned, plus they ask you if your mind has changed towards the person since your completion.

I had to admit I did get some things out of it. At the very beginning I was going to leave Sonita once I finished because of the unjust treatment she's been giving me. I knew I was innocent. Plus, I hate the fact that she could lie on me at any time and I'll be put away. That all changed and I realized <u>marriage</u> is a permanent growing process. Where you can't give up, give out, or give in. For better or for worse, just put that woman first, and pray to God to help it work. That's all you could do. So, with that in mind I was trying to handle our ups and downs. I wasn't going any where. My goal was to make the best of it. Communicate more. I came home to share with Sonita my last day and what I learned.

When I got home, no one was there.

My studio was torn up, papers were everywhere, my laptop was missing and no food was cooked. I'm thinking what happened now? Did Jerrica do this and Sonita left it like this for me to see or did Sonita do this. If so, why? What did I do now?

I called around but her family hadn't heard from her.

Finally, two hours later, she comes home with the family.

The family looks fine, but I can see she's mad.

I asked her, "What's up Bay? Why is upstairs torn up like this?"

She said," Hold on Love let me get the boys and Jerrica out the way."

I said," They fine, talk to me and where is my laptop?"

In the meantime we are taking off their coats and laying them down. I can tell they were tired.

Jerrica took it down and finally we are talking.

She said," Love I'm a ask you a question and I want a straight answer o.k.?"

I said,"Sonita I ask a question first, why is my stuff torn up?"

She said," Are you cheating on me?"

I said," What?"

She continued," Just answer are you?"

I screamed out, "No! What did you find or heard now! You been going through my things again haven't you?"

She replied," So what if I did. You're my husband, it's nothing you should be hiding from me anyway. I feel comfortable going through any thing of yours, you're mine!"

I said,"Sonita you got this relationship twisted. I don't go through your stuff out of respect for you as a person. I don't feel I got a right to violate your privacy with my curiosity."

She said, "I don't care! Who is Collin huh huh?

Who is she? I'm sitting here pregnant with your baby, and you writing Collin a letter stating you can't wait to come over her house. You aint shit! That's why your stuff is fucked up. Here take your little note."

She throws it at me and I pick it up and read it.

I said, "Sonita, Collin is a dude, he's selling me a guitar and a keyboard. I got to go to his house to check it out. Once I get it my music will sound much better. You torn up my shit on an assumption? You're gonna clean that shit up yourself.

I can't believe you I couldn't wait to get home, so I can tell you how my day was and this is what you do to me. I'm out!"

She sadly said," I'm sorry Love I didn't know, I thought you was cheating on me, please don't leave! Don't go! I'm sorry!"

I said," No, I'm out." I left and went to the go go bar and got drunk.

I got home around three in the morning. Sonita was upstairs crying cleaning up the last bit of stuff she tore up.

She wanted to talk but my head was spinning I just wanted to go to sleep. She wouldn't let me. Then I screamed at her by the top of my lungs," Leave me the fuck alone!"

That scared her and it work she left me alone.

The next day we talked. She was crying, I asked her,

"What's wrong?"

She said," I know your gonna leave me now."

I said," No I'm not, you haven't gave me a reason."

She sobbed and said," Well after I tell you this, you will."

I curiously asked, "What, the baby aint mine?"

She yelled out," No! you know this is your baby."

I sarcastically said," I don't know nothing now a days, I thought I knew you, but you seem to change day by day."

She paused and said," Well Love, I broke your laptop, I was mad at you and I wasn't thinking."

In denial I asked, "Sonita I know you are joking right? Right?" She started crying more. My heart drop and I fell to the floor. I continued, "It's no way you would do that. You know I got both of my movies type in there. Plus over 400 songs I wrote and ten years of my life recorded in there. How could you take my life away from me that stuff was gonna benefit us! Sonita us!

Our family, my other children, aaaahh this can't be happening!"

She said, "I'll buy you another one."

I screamed out, "Another one? I don't want another one, I want that one.!"

I left and went to work steamed!

I came home and tried to bring myself to talk to her, but it wouldn't work.

Sonita tried many times to talk with me but I went to sleep.

In the meantime, her stomached was getting big and her due date was right around the corner. I wasn't showing her any attention.

I would play with my sons and kick it with Jerrica. If Sonita asked me something I would give her short answers.

I was very disappointed with her. All that work I did on the lap top was gone. I didn't save anything on a disc or floppy. Sonita could tell I was hurt. She did everything in her power to make up with me.

However, I was at the end of my rope.

Then, on March 3, 2002, her water broke and I rushed her to the hospital. All the madness left me at that time and I was concerned about her and the baby. They had to induce her labor and three hours later Shereef was born on her third push.

He started crying and I said "Hey son, cut that out."

The nurse was surprised when he straighten up and looked at me.

The nurse said "Its amazing how he knows your voice."

I told her," I used to talk to him through her belly."

Then Sonita wanted to see him. Afterwards she went to sleep.

I went out in the hallway and told Jerrica Shereef was born.

Sonita sister had Jehdiah and Abijah. So I had to leave and get them. I was very happy my son was healthy and handsome.

Three days later they came home from the hospital.

Everything was fine. Both of our family members came through that week. Shereef looked like Jehdiah and Abijah put together.

Jehdiah and Abijah were very helpful and protective of their little brother. They would get the pampers, wipes, and his bottle for us. That way Sonita could rest. I continued to work and take care of the family. Sonita wouldn't let Jerrica hold or touch Shereef.

She decided in two months she would get a job.

My brother Ibn came down for my birthday and to see my son.

We partied.

It was Sonita, Ibn, Kiesha, Shah, Samad, Jan and me.

We celebrated my birthday and the birth of Shereef.

All the fellas went to the bar, played pool and drank.

The ladies stayed home, played cards and talked.

When we came home, then the party got liver.

We had so much fun.

In April, her cousin went to Atlanta and told her, "Atlanta would be a good place to live." Sonita wanted to give it a shot.

Sonita really didn't want to stay in V.A. I told her,

"My sister and cousin are in Atlanta, so if you want to make that move we can go.

Visit them first, then put a plan together to reach it."

She said," Word, Love, I'm with it."

We put that plan in effect for the near future.

In the mean time, we dealt with our children and Jerrica.

Jehdiah and Abijah would go at it playing in house basketball.

Jehdiah was nice, he would try to do the moves he saw on my an one tapes. When he would drive to the hole his favorite line was,

"What you're gonna do ,what you're gonna do? "

Then he would take his shot and make it.

Abijah didn't like it so he would try to fight Jehdiah.

Afterwards Jehdiah would laugh and run from him.

Once Abijah got the ball he would throw it at the door.

He really didn't care to make the shot, if it hit the door he was cool.

Shereef would sit in his swinger and just watch.

Sonita and I would just be laughing our tail off.

Jerrica would watch and trip off our sons too.

There was an abundance of peace, love, and happiness in the air.

People felt it when they came into our home.

Then, one day Jerrica didn't get off the bus. Sonita called me at work and said, "Jerrica isn't home." I was sick I didn't know what to do. I left work and went looking for her. We called the cops and made a report. Three hours later, I find her at this complex where Sonita said she might be.

When I rode up on her she was riding a bike. Upon spotting me and coming up on her, she broke started running and began screaming. The little kids were telling her, "Keep running, keep running!" We went through backyards and alley ways, but I finally caught her. I asked her, "What the hell was you thinking?

Why did you make me chase you?

You know your ass is getting whipped. Now get in the car."

She screamed out, "I don't want a beating I want to live with my friends!"

I said, "The only place your gonna live is with us. Other than that, the system will put you away."

I took her home and whipped her tail. I called the cops to let them know I found her. We put her on punishment and made her read.

May came around and Jerrica ran away again. This time she was gone for 8 hours. I get a call from the cops saying they found her at a different complex about to go into this apartment with a man. Once the officer said her name, she turned around and the guy left and went inside the building.

I put her on punishment again. Sonita was vexed by now.

She could clearly see Jerrica was taking advantage of my sympathy for her. Sonita told her," If you run away again, you are going back to New Jersey."

It wasn't even two weeks before Jerrica ran away again.

This time she was gone for three days. If it weren't for the lady being suspicious about Jerrica story we probably wouldn't a found her.

After that time Sonita said, "Love, your cousin got to go. I don't want her here."

I was crushed there was nothing I could do, Jerrica wasn't really listening to me from Sonita's stand point.

Therefore in June I took Jerrica back to Newark New Jersey to the system. Then, I left.

It hurt me to my heart that I couldn't do more for her.

Once I got back home Sonita and I started contacting my cousin and sister to set up our first trip down there.

In the meantime, I'm renting out studio time and making a little extra money. I had 10 songs of my own done by myself.

Jehdiah loved Sesame Street, and The Learning Channel.

He always used to say, "When can I go to my school?"

We were so happy to see how interested he was in attending school. He was only four, however he wanted to go to school since he was two.

Abijah didn't want to do nothing but be under us. When they attended the summer head start program at James Monroe Abijah would cry when we left. He didn't listen to any of the teachers. Only Jehdiah could make him sit down and do his work. We would drop them off and pick them up together, whenever my schedule allowed.

I went on the field trips with them while Sonita took care of Shereef. Teamwork was our thing with our sons.

Now that Jerrica was gone, they received a lot of attention, love, and extra time.

Sonita tells me, "Love, I'm pregnant again."

I asked her," Are you sure?"

She said, "Yes Love, I 'm having the same symptoms as before."

Later on we went to the doctors and she was right. We were having another one and Shereef wasn't even one year old yet.

The nurse told us," Be very careful because a women body needs a year to heal from having a baby, however Sonita body hasn't healed yet. It is going through changes now. You probably feel more depress than usual; little things that never bothered you will bother you now because of the chemical unbalance of your hormones.

You're going to need a lot of rest this pregnancy because you're going through a high risk pregnancy."

When we left Sonita started crying. I was puzzled.

I asked her, "What's wrong?"

She softly said, "Love, everything she said, is the way I feel. I just didn't know how to tell you. That's why I wanted the day hours, so I could rest and get up when the boys get up." I said to her,

"Sonita I'm gonna be there for you the whole step of the way.

You will get better."

Now, we knew we had to really save our money so we could go to Atlanta to prepare a better life for our children.

We moved out of the condo in July to a one- bedroom apartment so we could save money and roll. We put the rest of our things into storage. There were some dudes who lived across from us. One of the dudes I knew from coming into the shop. The rest of his friends I had just met.

One dude was selling mixed c.d.s He would always seem to catch me whenever I got off from work. I could see they were sweating my wife. However when I'm around they play their part. Our neighbors were cool. We actually moved closer to Sonita job and further from mine.

The Summer Head Start Program was over in August and it was time for me to enroll Jehdiah in Stuart Early Child Development Center. I enrolled Jehdiah in school, and his moms attended the Teachers and Parents Conference.

Jehdiah was so happy to know he was going to school.

That's all he talked about.

Sonita kept complaining about her back. Sometimes she would just cry from the pain. I'll rub it or make love to her and she would sleep like a bird.

One day I ran into Danielle; she sings. The last time I heard her sing was 1999. She needed work although she had heart.

I gave her my c.d. and I told her to listen to it.

Sam does beats and he would come to the shop and let me here them. One of the beats I fell in love with. I invited him to the studio. He and I got along good and it wasn't long before we had three songs together.

Sonita's job still wouldn't change her schedule. That was bothering her a lot. So my sons and I would ride her to work and pick her up. Other times she would drive herself.

One day we were watching videos and Musiq video came on.

I sung it to her, *"I will Love you when your hair turn gray girl,"*
I will love you if you gain a little weight girl"

She started blushing. I hugged her and kissed her. Jehdiah and Abijah were watching. They jumped up between us and we held the both of them. Shereef started pushing himself over to us.

We pulled him out of his walker and held him as well. Then, we tickled all three of them. They were laughing at the top of their lungs. Afterwards, we fed them and took it down.

The next week we went clothes shopping for Jehdiah.

School was right around the corner and we wanted to be prepared.

Sonita was so happy her son was going to school. She kept saying, "I'm a be there on his first day of school."

Abijah would start school the following year.

Shereef was moving fast. There was no place he couldn't get to in his walker. We knew from his actions that he was moving out of the way for the next baby.

September came and Sonita still had the grave yard shift.

She was complaining about her body because she wasn't getting enough rest. When I leave to go to work, she's coming in and the boys would be up. I'll make them breakfast and put in a movie for them to watch. Abijah knew how to take the tape out and change it. He and Shereef would watch the two movies that way Sonita could sleep. It gave her four hours of undisturbed sleep. However, if Abijah or Shereef became hungry or agitated they would wake her up from sleep.

September 2, 2002 was the first day of school for Jehdiah and Sonita was too tired to take him.

I took pictures of him at the house. Jehdiah was so happy. Sonita gave him a hugg then a kiss and off we went.

I arrived to the school a little early. We were outside with the other parents and kids. Jehdiah and I recognized some people who came into the barbershop. We talked until they let us in. I looked for the gold room so I could find his teacher. Kids and people were everywhere.

I found his teacher and I introduced him to her. He was so cool about everything. Other kids were coming up to him as I was taking pictures of him. When the kids wanted to shake his hand he would pull them close to him like I do and pat them on their back. Other kids were looking on and before long he had the other children imitating him. Right then I knew he was a star.

I just smiled and looked on.

Before long Jehdiah said, "You can go daddy, I'm cool."

I said," What, are you alright?"

He said "Yes, dad bye."(smile)

I was shocked. I figured he would want me to walk him to his class. He was totally comfortable with the environment.

I said," Okay. son I'm out. I'll pick you up later, right over here."
He said,"O k. dad."

I started walking towards the door, talking to different parents on my way out. I kept looking back at Jehdiah to see if he was paying any attention to me leaving and he wasn't.

I was so proud of him. Eventually I left and went to work.

I told the fellas at the barbershop about my son, and how cool he was on his first day.

I went back and pick him up from school. He was cheezing.

His teacher said he was good and she couldn't wait to see him the next day.

I took him to McDonalds and bought him and the family something to eat.

Once we got home I told Sonita about his first day.

Jehdiah gave her the papers from his teacher and Sonita read them smiling I left and went back to work.

When I finished working I went straight home.

Sonita and I talked about her day with the boys.

Sonita said, "Abijah and Shereef woke me up saying eat, eat. So I got up and fed them; then I went back to sleep."

I said," Word, so are you alright?"

She said," Yes I'm good. Your dinner is in the oven."

I said, "Thanks baby."

As I ate Sonita put on Angie Stone album.

She said, "Listen to this song, I love it."

The song was, *I rather be facing 25 to life,*

If I can't be your wife.

She put it on repeat and played it until she had to go to work.

I said, "That's a crazy love song, it's nice though, for real Sonita."

This was how Jehdiah's first week went at school.

It only changed if Sonita had a day off, then she would take him.

Whenever she came back from taking him, she would talk about how bright Jehdiah was.

On September 9, 2002, I started attending barber school at night, on Mondays and Wednesdays.

I took Jehdiah to school the second week.

I drove myself to school Monday and Sonita took me Wednesday.

In the meantime, Spoon started calling me so I could work on some songs. Sam was down with going to the studio. I got in contact with Danielle and Indoe and they both wanted to be there. Therefore I planned it for the following Monday on September 16, 2002.

I mentioned it to Sonita on September 12, 2002.

She was fine with it.

Over the weekend Sonita is having crazy mood swings.

She started crying for no reason again.

Sonita stopped doing the routine we established for Jehdiah and me going to school.

She would tell me, "Love, I don't get that much sleep and my back be hurting. I wish this pain would go away. I can't take no medicine because I'm pregnant. You did this to me!

I wish you could feel this pain just one time!"

I said, "How is it my fault you wanted to do it. If I say no to you, you swear I've been cheating on you."

She said," What ever Love, I have a doctor's appointment in two weeks on September 24; are you going with me?"

I said," Yes, Sonita as long as it falls on a slow day at the barbershop."

She said," I know, I know, it is on your slow day."

Sunday September 15, We all watched a movie together. I worked on some of my music. Jehdiah, Abijah, and Shereef are playing together. Sonita was happy, talking on the phone to her family.

We ate dinner and talked a little before we went to bed.

On September 16, 2002, Sonita woke up from Shereef's crying.

Afterwards the boys followed. I was the last to get up. It was heavy rain and hurricane winds in the forecast. While Sonita is tending to Shereef I'm looking for my clothes. I see the time and I'm running behind to pick everybody up to go to the studio.

Jehdiah and Abijah are playing basketball now.

I said, "Sonita I'm a see you before I go to school."

She asked," Where are you going?"

I said, "To the studio, remember I told you last week I was going Monday."

She said, "I didn't know it was today. Cancel out, this is my day off, I want to spend it with you. We need to talk Bay."

I said," I can't cancel it, everybody is waiting for me to pick them up.

Its only for three hours. We are doing just vocals."

She said, "Forget that Love, that can wait, I really need to talk to you about what's been on my mind."

I said,"Sonita we will do that when I'm finished, I'm out."

I went to the door. Sonita put Shereef down and followed me down the stairs. Our apartment door is open and the boys are in the living room by the door.

I'm walking to the car and Sonita shouts.

"You care about your music more than you care about me!"

I yelled back," No, I don't Sonita, You know better. Calm down and don't make a scene out here. I promise you I'll be right back we will talk then."

Now, I'm inside the car about to shut the door and she rushed me and scratched me on my neck.

She screamed again," You don't love me you don't care.!!"

I said," Whatever Sonita, are you happy, my neck is bleeding now."

I pushed her off me then I slammed the door. I rolled down the window a little and scream out." Your ass need some help!

Get back in the house I can hear Jehdiah on the steps calling Shereef name!"

She said, "What do you care, your going to the studio any way!

If you pull off, Love I'm a break up your shit!"

I said, "I love you anyway, bye Sonita."

I pulled off and had to think fast. Sam and Danielle lived within 5 minutes of each other. Indoe lived about 15 minutes away from me and an extra 20 minutes away from them. I decided to just pick up Danielle and Sam. Sam had the beat and Danielle is gonna sing the hook. The song is about Sonita and I. *My Homey Lovin Friend.*

We got to Spoon's house about an half a hour late. He was cool with it and we started the session. It went longer than we expected, but we got it done. During the last mix down we heard thunder and lightening. It was raining very hard. Floods were everywhere. Sam had to be at work by 4:30pm he worked at Blockbusters on 21street in Norfolk. I had to be to school by 6:00pm and It was 4:00pm when we left. I couldn't find a clear path any where.

It was backed up. Cars were floating while others were stuck.

In the mist of getting Sam to work, Danielle asked me, "Who was the song about?"

I happily replied, "My wife Sonita. This is how it was for us back in the day."

I got Sam to work at 4:53pm. I drop Danielle off at 5:00pm.

I headed home to Sonita. I got there at 5:30pm. Water was inside the car. When I put my key in the door to turn the knob, the door wouldn't open. I had to push the door open. Jehdiah, Abijah, and Shereef were watching television my computer, printer, vcr, and radio was broke. My clothes was piled up at the door.

I just put my head down I was crushed. I knew she was probably mad because I was late. But I figured, if I let her hear the completed copy she would understand. I couldn't do that, though, because she broke my radio.

Sonita came out the bedroom looking shocked. She didn't hear me come in. When she saw me, she ran back into the room.

I didn't even bother to chase her. I just picked up my things and took them to the car. She came out the room and said.

"Give me my key I don't want you here."

After I put my last things in the car I gave her the key.

She started crying I didn't show no emotions. However she could tell I was hurt. I couldn't go to school because it was 6:30pm when I finished. I had no where to go, so I rode to Indoe house.

I told him, "Its raining like crazy and Sonita just put me out the house. "

TWELVE
The Unthinkable

INDOE SAID," WORD THAT'S fucked up. What happened to you earlier?"

I told him, "Sonita held me up and I was running late so I picked up Sam and Danielle and went. My bad."

He said,"Alright, well I got a forty do you wants some?"

I said "Yeah."

I drank up his beer, then I went to Samad's house and told him what had happen. He fed me, then we went to the go go bar and played pool. Afterwards, I left, rode back to my house and slept in my car through the pouring rain.

September 17, 2002, Tuesday morning. I knock on the door and she opened it, Jehdiah was happy to see me, he was ready to go to school. She couldn't find his sneakers. Jehdiah and I found them under the couch, then we left.

After I dropped him off I went to my job and slept in the parkinlot until some one came.

After school I pick him up and took him home. Abijah and Shereef were watching TV. The house was messy. I told her," You need to clean up."

She said," Don't worry about it, you don't live here."

I said," Whatever Sonita."

She continued, "Look I got a baby sitter for the boys. I need you to take me to work and drop me off."

"O.k. I'll be back by 10:30."

I left and went to Sam's house. I told him "I liked the song."

He told me "Danielle wanted to do her vocals over."

I said, "I'm a book some more time, and we will work on it."

I left from his house and went to take her to work.

I slept in the car again then I picked her up September 18, 2002 Wednesday morning. She had to go to Chesapeake to pick the children up. I stayed home though. Sonita took Jehdiah to school. Then she came home with Abijah and Shereef. I left and went to work. I get a call from Vernon. He said,

"Yo dog it's on and popping. I'm here and I need a cut, so what's up?"

I said, "Word Vernon, no bullshit are you here?"

He excitedly said, "Yeah, I'm with Melvin now, we are coming to the shop."

I was so happy because Vernon was like a big brother to me. Ever since I was small. Everywhere I been he always stayed in contact with me. If he had it, it was mine.

His younger brother Bruce was my older brother Dawoo's best friend. They used to wild out together in the heart of all trouble. Vernon moved to Hawaii, and still stayed in contact with me. I chilled with Melvin and him at Melvin's house.

I told him my situation with Sonita.

I said, "Look Vernon this is the fourth time she's thrown me out for nothing. Shit, I might as well get some pussy as much as I been accused of cheating." He said,

"No Love, just continue doing what you're doing. Bust that school out so you can get your barber's license. That way you can go anywhere and cut. You can move to Hawaii for real and be alright." I said,

"Yeah, I bet, but first I'm getting my own place. I'm tired of living like this Vernon. I can't even invite you over to my place. You know why, I don't have a place! My first week of school and we are beefing!

Now my second week of school, I'm homeless!

I can't miss three days or I'll automatically fail." Tears are falling down my face. He said,

"Love, you got to understand, Sonita is young and she's pregnant again. Things a work out with ya'll, just give her some space."

I said, "Fuck that, what about my space, I'm not going back to her, I'm a get my own and deal with her from afar!"

Vernon continued, "Love I know its tough, look at me and Leqeitha. We been married for 18 years now and I took her through a world of shit.

We've been separated one time for a whole year and we got back together and made it. You can do it too." I said,

"I hear you Vernon, but it's not fair that I got to go through life like this. I'm not sleeping in the streets all my life. I'm a get me a roof over my head." He said,

"You don't need too, just go back to Sonita and talk about it.

You know she's gonna need your help with those three boys.

Stay with her Love, just deal with it."

I said, "Whatever man."

We kicked it for another hour, then he left to sleep in his hotel room, while I slept in my car.

September 19, 2002, Thursday I went home to take Jehdiah to school. She was running behind so I dropped Jehdiah off and circled back to feed Abijah and Shereef.

Afterwards I went to work.

Around 2:00pm Sonita came to my job saying,

"I need the car."

I said, "Okay, let me get my things out the car first."

She said, "Go ahead."

I went back into the barbershop and asked Pat could I put my things in his trunk until later. I really didn't want anyone to know what I was going through but I had no choice.

After I put my things in his trunk, she was mad. She said,

"Oh you're letting everyone know our business huh?"

I said, "You're the one who came here to take the car from me. You know I don't have any other means."

She said, "Well you got your things bye."

I said, "Bye."

I went back into the shop explaining my life because everyone was watching.

That night I asked Pat could I sleep in the new shop he was getting. It was an old car repair shop that had mice in there and everything. I didn't care I needed somewhere to sleep. He said, "Yeah." I slept there that night.

September 20, 2002, Friday. I went to Donut Dinette for breakfast, afterwards I went in to work. Now, Sonita has to take Jehdiah to school.

She didn't get any sleep. Abijah and Shereef were bothering her because I'd usually pull out two movies and Abijah knew what to do from there. Sonita came home from work and went to sleep. They wouldn't let her. The normal four hours she would have was gone She had to do everything herself.

Around 4:00pm The shop door opened. It was Jehdiah.

He said, "Mommy want you daddy."

I said, "Okay son, tell her I'm coming."

I told my client I'll be a minute.

Mink said," Yeah right."

I told him, "Watch you'll see Mink."

I went outside and Shereef and Abijah face's lit up. They both were trying to get out. I open the doors and let them out. I hugged and kissed them.

Sonita spoke. "Where is my kiss?"

I hugged and kissed her two. The boys just laughed.

I said, "So what's up Sonita, how are you?"

She responded with, "I'm find and maintaining. Look Love are you still going with me to my appointment Tuesday?"

I told her, "Yes, I said I will."

She continued, "O.k. well we are hungry I need some money. Smile I said, "I knew that was coming, how much?"

She softly said, "Just ten dollars would do. Jehdiah was real good today. His teacher loves him."

I said, "That's my boy, keep up the good work son."

Jehdiah said, "Yes sir!" smile, he then saluted me like a soldier.

Sonita was amazed, she looked at me with confusion in her eyes.

She said, "Where did he get that from?"

I said, "From the military movies I watched. You know he will stay up with me after you fall asleep."

She continued, "Alright Love we are out. I'll call you."

I screamed out, "Bye boys!"

Abijah screamed back, "Give me kiss, give me kiss."

So I kissed them all again and they left.

I went back inside and finished cutting.

At the end of the night I slept in the shop again.

Saturday I went and looked for me a room in the hood.

I found a spot on w 41street in Norfolk, however I wouldn't be able to move in until next Saturday. I had to find me a place to sleep tonight because Pat's construction workers was pulling an all nighter. I called around to a couple of people but nothing seemed promising. After work I went to a bar and got drunk.

Then I went to Grandy Park and went to sleep.

Sunday I went to Sam's house to check him. He told me,

"Danielle came over yesterday, we listen to the song and played some games." I said,

"Word that's good, keep her on point, she got the look we just need her to bust out her vocals." Sam said,

"Oh, I got that under control. She's gonna be nice when I finish with her."

His moms cooked dinner and it was banging. I told her,

"I haven't had cooking like this since my mother died. smile She just laughed and told me, "Come over anytime."

I said, "You got it."

I left and got drunk by myself in the park. I started reminiscing on my life. As I went back in my mind it hit me like a ton of bricks. YOU DON'T HAVE NOBODY. 80% of my family is DEAD. Why am I still here? What is my purpose? I have another failed marriage. Nobody loves me or even cares.

Before I knew it, I was crying my heart out in Grandy Park.

Afterwards I fell to sleep.

Monday, September 23, 2002, I went to eat at McDonalds. I stayed in there for two hours thinking over, where can I go? Something pop in my head.

Let me make sure Mitch is still holding my room.

He was home and he reassured me, he would hold it.

When I left him, I walked to Jehdiah's school to see him get out.

When he saw me, he was surprised and happy. We played basketball on the playground. Just him and I. Sonita came shortly after and he didn't want to go. However I encouraged him to go on. I waved bye and she pulled off. I stayed on the playground for a while, to my surprise Sonita pulled up.

She said, "Love get in, I want to talk to you."

I got in and we rode around talking. She said,

"Love it's hard getting the boys together by myself.

I got to pick the kids up from Chesapeake and ride all the way home, change Jehdiah's clothes, take him to school, then tend to Abijah and Shereef." I said to her,

"Well you brought that on yourself, you put me out and took the car away from me." She said,

"I know Bay, I know. Could you watch them for me at night and you could go to work from here?" I said,

"I'm not with it. You think you can just throw me out when you want, then let me stay there to benefit you! In the meantime I still don't have a place to stay. For what? I was doing a song about us and this is what I get. I'm a find me a place and get on my feet. Then we can switch with the kids." She said,

"I'm a need some money for the babysitter then." I told her,

"I don't have none. Maybe Saturday I'll have something for you."
She asked,

"Okay that's fine, I'm off Saturday, I'll check you at your job.
Where do you want me to drop you off at?"

I said, "Out in Park Place by the shop."

We rode around for a little while longer, then she dropped me off.

I went to Sam's house and crashed over there.

Tuesday September 24, 2002, I went to work and it was slow.

Around 1:00pm Sonita picked me up and we went to her appointment.

I stayed out in the lobby with our children while Sonita went in the room to be checked. I read a couple of pamphlets, then I attended to the boys. 20 minutes later, Sonita came out with the nurse. Sonita introduced her to me and the children. The receptionist complimented us on how good our children were in the waiting room. The nurse told us then, Sonita's due date was on April 25, 2003; we were very happy about this. That was the day we got married. The nurse gave Sonita some brochures and she instructed me, "Make sure Sonita do light work. This pregnancy will be tough on her."

We left and went back to her place.

There we put in a movie for the boys and we went into the room to talk. She said,

"Love I'm a ask you a question, and just be honest."

I said, "O lord, here we go again. What's up now?"

She said," I'm not accusing you of nothing, I just want the truth."

I said, "Okay what is it?"

She sadly said," If I die, would you remarry?"

With shock and concern I said, "What? Are you crazy?
What do you mean if you die.
What's wrong with you? What did the doctor say? You might die having birth or something?" She said,

"No Bay, but I be having some crazy thoughts. I mean, I can't even bring myself to tell you what's be running through my mind. I'm tired Love for real. Sometimes I don't want to get up."

I softly said, "Sonita listen. I love you more than life itself. I'd probably die before you the way the statistics goes for Black men. So don't think about something so cruel. How do you think our sons would be if you leave us; and as far as your answer. No! I wont marry no one else. I rather die and see you in the new system.

Than to live the rest of my life with another woman."

Sonita started crying and I held her in my arms and cried with her. I said,

"Sonita I don't know why you do these thing to me. Or why I do these things to you. Like we don't have any feelings. I want to be with you, but you put me out. So eventually I'm getting me a place one day." She said,

"Why, when you can move back in with me. I'm sorry Love for real I wasn't thinking I need you here."

I really wanted to stay and give in but my pride wouldn't let me.

We started kissing and we made love. As soon as she climax she burst out in tears, crying harder than I ever witnessed before.

I asked her, "What's wrong with you Sonita? Why are you crying so hard?" She sadly said,

"Just take the key please, I want you to stay, in a crying tone I told her, "I'm about to go to work, I don't need the key, bye."

She cried and said, "O.k, O.k Love, I understand your gonna get your own." Then I said,

"I'm still gonna take care of our sons, and you. I got to go to work now. We are gonna have another baby on our anniversary!"

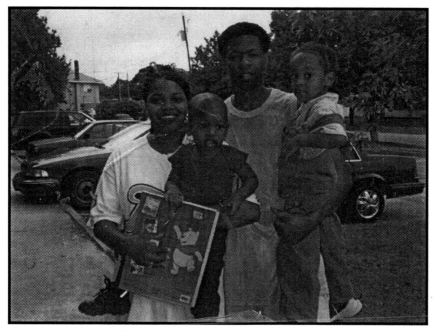

Sonita, Abijah, Randell, and Jehdiah, in front of our home.

I went back to work and finished cutting.

I left to pick Jehdiah up from school and he told me how his day went, and I took him home. Sonita was up by then, so she dropped me back off at the shop. She told me," I'll bring the boys by tomorrow to see you after school." I said,

"That's peace, bye ya'll! I'm waving at this time.

Waving back, my sons screamed out," Bye daddy! Bye!

I go back inside and grind for the rest of the day.

Sonita was on my mind. Everything we discussed was running through my head. I really wanted to give in, but my pride was in the way. I wanted to teach her a lesson. You can't just throw me out and expect me to come back to you like its cool.

I was getting me a spot simply because if we beef I won't have to be in the streets like I'm living now. Matter of fact I have to find a place to stay tonight. Pat's construction workers were pulling an all nighter. I had to find me another place for the night.

Sam popped in my head. I'll check him tonight.

I got to his house about 9:30pm. His mom offered me something to eat. While I was eating she schooled me on how women can act.

I really appreciated her conversation. It gave me a different way to view things.

I talked with Sam, afterwards, and then I left. I really didn't want to impose another night. During my walk through Park Place I ran into my client named Bryant. He screamed out,

"You need a ride?"

I said, "Yeah pull over!"

I got in and told him." Take me to Sabrina's house."

He said, "That's the girl who stays over by Grandy?"

I said, "Word."

I brief him on my situation on the way.

Bryant listened and said, "I wish I had a spot for you ace, but I'm out back myself."

I said, "I understand fam, Im a survive though."

He replied, "Oh no doubt, I know you'll be alright. Just keep your head up."

Sabrina was home so he bounced. I told her what was going on and she let me crash on her couch. I slept like a bird.

Wednesday, September 25, 2002, I left Sabrina's house and went to the shop. Everybody knew I wasn't home with my wife because I had the same clothes on. I worked and kept to myself, thinking constantly over my life. Around 4:00pm Jehdiah came in the shop.

He said, "Daddy mommy wants you." (Smile)

I said, "O.K. son tell her I'm coming."

I went outside and Sonita was smiling from ear to ear.

I spoke, "Hey family!" Abijah and Shereef are smiling so I tickle them and they burst out laughing.

I asked, "So what's up Sonita?"

She said,"Oh nothing, I told you I would bring the boys by to see you."

I said, "That was thoughtful, what's going on with you?"

She replied, "The same old same, I'm finally getting the hang at putting two movies out for Abijah. He loves Spiderman and Training Day.

I woke up to Shereef's crying. He had stinked on himself and he was hungry. I fed him and Abijah and they were fine. I told my manager to switch me off of the graveyard shift so I could rest better. But this chick still has'nt done it. I'm about to go over her head."

I replied, "Well baby, do what you got to do."

She looked at me and said,

"Love I know you're at work so I'll call you or come by tomorrow."

I said, "Alright talk to you later."

They left. I went inside and finish cutting. Moe came in to get his haircut from Mink. He invited us over to his house to play pool.

We were all for it, however when the time came, Mink changed his mind. I ended up going by myself. As a result.

I had a ball with Moe and his friends. I asked Moe could I spend the night. He said, "Yeah, but I had to leave in the morning."

Thursday September 26, 2002, it was a beautiful morning.

The sun was out and it was hot. I decided to walk to Donut Dinette for breakfast. Moe lived on Golsnin and 37street.

I figured I'll walk down Godsnold to 25street and turn on to Colley. Then I walked straight down to 21street. I ate and left to go to 7 Eleven on 20street. Soon as I got there, something told me to turn around. Once I did, I saw Sonita and my sons pulling up. I walked out of the store and said, "How did you find me?"

She said, "I rode around by your job and went on instinct to see if you ate at Donut Dinette. Jehdiah spotted you first and once I looked I knew it was you."(Smile)

I asked her," What's on your mind?"

She replied, "I couldn't sleep last night, you was on my mind, so I set out to find you to talk." I said,

"Okay, let me get something to drink and I'll get in.

Do you need anything?"

She smiled and said, "No I'm fine."

I went inside, got the boys some sweets and me something to drink. I got in the car and we rode around for awhile talking.

Sonita said, "Love my manager is taking forever to change my schedule so I'm a cut back on my hours. I don't know what's been going on with me lately. I can tell you're still upset with me by the way we talked on the phone. I don't want to lose you. The boys miss you and it's tough on me. I'm really sorry for putting you out." Again I said,

"I believe you Sonita and I'm sorry too for not staying home that Monday and just hearing you out. I wish I could take that day back. You really hurt my feelings. I love you and I want to make it work. But what's gonna happen when you get mad at me again? Are you gonna throw me out? These thoughts plagued my mind. In the meantime she is pulling up on the side of the barbershop.

I sadly responded," I can't live like this Sonita."

While tears are falling down her eyes she said," I know love.

I just lost my grandfather two years ago and you are all I have left.

I'm even willing to go through a marriage counselor to show you I'm trying to do better."

I said," You can if you want to, I been through enough counseling with anger management."

She asked me, "Well, will you come home?"

I told her, "Yes Sonita I will. I miss ya'll so much; I'm tired of being in these streets."

We hugged and kissed.

Sonita said, "Love it's about time for Jehdiah to go to school. I'm a drop him off and go home to get some rest."

I said, "O.k. I'm a wait out here for the barbershop to open. Just swing back bye after school so I could see ya'll."

I hugged and kissed the boys, and then I walked over to stand in front of the shop. Sonita pulled off.

Next door to the barbershop was a Salon. The lady who own's it was in there. I waved and she waved for me to come inside.

I did and said, "Hi Lynn,"

She responded, "Hi Love. That was your wife you was talking to?"

I said, "Yeah, we are going through some things. She's on her way to take my son to school."

Then she said, "Yeah, what school do he go to?"

I replied, "Stuart."

She said," Really, I hear it's a good school."

I continued," Word, one of my clients put me up on it. My son love it too."

In the mist of our conversation Sonita pulled back up.

My heart jumped. I was scared because I know Sonita doesn't like me talking to women. I walked out side and spoke,

"What's up Bay?" She shouted,

"Don't what's up me, why are you in there talking to that bitch! You want her or something? Is that's why you wanted to wait out here so you can talk to her huh, huh?" I said,

"No Sonita you got it all wrong we were just talking about the school Jehdiah go to." Sonita said,

"I don't want to hear that shit, you know what, I'm a go ahead and do what I was thinking to do." I curiously asked,

"What's that, take me to court for custody or something?"

She said, "No you're a see watch. I'm a go in there and fuck her up." I stood in front of her and nervously said,

"See Sonita that's uncall for. Please don't make a scene.

While we are talking Pat pulls up and some clients are behind him. I continued,

"I wont talk to her no more okay, You is who I want for real. We just said we were going to work on our relationship right?"

She said, "Right, but I haven't left you for ten minutes and your already up in another woman's face!"

Pat speaks and so does his client. One of them name Mark waved for me to come here.

I told her, "Sonita I'll be right back, just chill out."

She smirked and said," Make it quick."

He showed me his car he was selling it was nice, but I knew I didn't have any dough to buy it so I walked back to Sonita and finished talking. I said,

"Look Sonita, this weekend I'll spend with ya'll and we can start back getting our lives together."

She smiled and said, "O.k. Love, but kiss me right now in front of her."

I asked "Why?"

She continued, "If you're not trying to talk to her, just do it."

I smiled and said," Okay Bay."

I told her, "Get out the car," and I hugged and kissed her in front of the shop so everybody could see. Sonita felt much better.

She said, "Now Love, don't let me catch you in her shop again."

I quickly said," You wont, I promise."

Afterwards Sonita left and went home. I didn't even look towards Lynn's shop I just walked in the barbershop and kick it with Pat and his clients.

I worked all day and at 4:00pm Jehdiah came in the shop.

He said, "Come out side daddy, mommy wants you."

I told him, "Here I come."

I went out side and kick it with her; she told me she needed some money to feed the kids so I gave her 20 dollars.

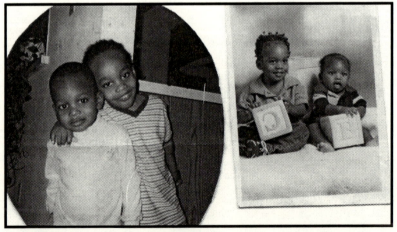

ABIJAH AND JEHDIAH, 2002 LEFT. 2000 RIGHT.

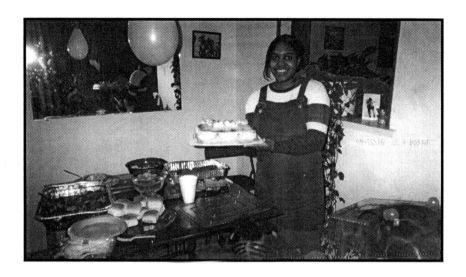

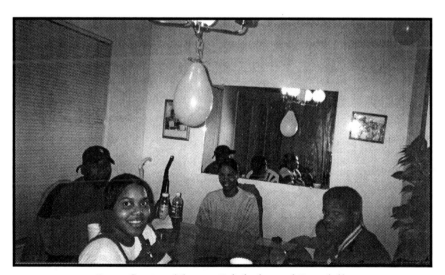

Jazz, Sonita, Teresa, Jehdiah, and Randell.
The top picture is Shereef's baby shower.

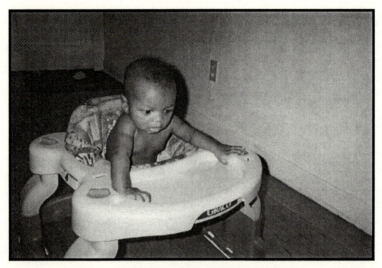

Shereef in his walker 7months old.

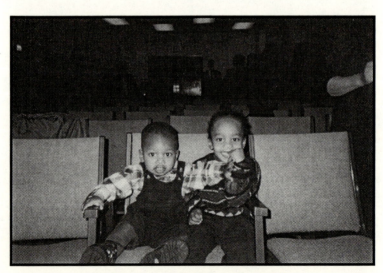

Abijah, and Jehdiah at the Hall

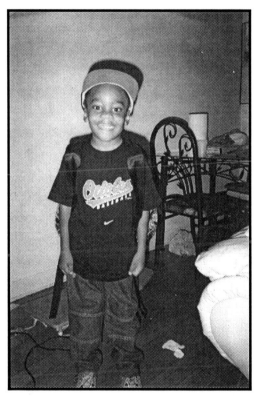

Jehdiah's first day of school, he was very happy.

She then asked me," Do you want me to bring you something back?"

I said, "Yeah whatever you can."

Sonita left and got some Hardees Chicken. I took two pieces and a biscuit out and she left.

At the end of the night I had to figure out where I was going to sleep. I'll ask Sam's mom if I could stay for the next two days. That way I could move into my room Saturday and be straight.

Therefore I went, got me a beer, and walked over to his house. His mom didn't mind. I listened to music all night with Sam and we took it down after that.

Friday September 27, 2002, I went to work and grind as usual.

Sonita came by with my sons. She looked tired.

She said, "Love you know rent is coming up are you gonna give me some money on it?" I told her,

"Yes, I'm a give you half and $50.00 toward the babysitter."

She said, "That's it? What about money for me?"

I told her,"Sonita I'm the one out here in these streets, I need money for myself. You work don't you? It's nothing else I can do."

She said, "But I got all the children though, your free to do what you want. You don't have any responsibilities! You're probably whoring around with these bitches while I'm struggling with the kids." I screamed out,

"No I'm not! You keep blaming me like I left you. YOU put me out!" Exasperated she said,

"You know what I don't want to argue no more. Just give me what you want; I'll get by some how. Oh and tell your friends to stop harassing me."

I curiously asked her," Who are you talking about?"

She said, "Them guys in the building across from us, every time they see me they try to push up on me. Sometimes they be staring at me through my window." I said,

"Word! Why are you telling me this now? I could've been step to them. One of them work at Donut Dinette. I'm a check him."

She said, "It's not him, but the other dudes who you brought the movies and c.ds from. If you were home with us I wouldn't have this problem." I said,

"Whatever Sonita Tomorrow is Saturday when I get off, I'll come spend the night with ya'll. I'll deal with it, plus I'll give you the money." She said,

"Well you can at least take me out to dinner?"

I said," I'll see"

She left after that and I went back inside and started cutting.

Mitch came through for the money for the room, but I told him I'll have it all Saturday. He said he would wait in the meantime he needed a haircut. As a favor, I hooked him up.

That night I slept over Sam's house again.

Saturday September 28, 2002. I went to work and it was packed.

I was glad because I needed everything I could make so I could pay everybody their money.

Mitch gave me until 6:00pm to pay. I called Samad and told him, "I'm a need your help to move my things in the room."

He said, "I'd would be available around 9:00pm. In the meantime, Sonita calls me around 3:00pm "Love, I'm a pick you up from work tonight." I told her,

"You don't have to, Samad is gonna drop me off to you when I get off."

She said, "When would that be?"

I said, "After 9:00pm then we can go out to eat dinner o.k."

She said,"Alright Love call me when your on your way."

6:00pm came and I went to pay Mitch for the room. He gave me the keys and I told him I'll be back around 9:00pm to move my things in. I paid Pat his money at 8:00pm. Samad came through around 9:00pm. We went to Sam's house and got all my things. It was taking longer than we expected so I called Sonita and told her,

"I'm running behind but, I'm still coming."

I can hear the kids in the background crying. She said,

"Never mind Love, I don't want to go out in eat, just come home the kids are stressing me out."

I asked her, "Why are you crying, what's wrong?"

Sobbing she said," I can't take it no more, just come home, it don't matter what time. Just come home please."

I sensed something was wrong; then I said, "Okay Sonita but listen if we aren't going out I'll be there in the morning around 10:00." She said,

"No Love, come tonight I don't care how late it is."

I told her,"Sonita I promise you I'll be there in the morning."

She dejected said, "Okay Love, Okay."

I knew I had to meet with Mitch and go over his rules and regulations concerning the rooming house. Plus, Samad had to do some things for his family. When that was all done it was 12:00am in the morning. I went to sleep in my bed and slept like a bird.

Sunday, September 29, 2002, I got up at 8:00am. I washed and got dressed. I went to the bus stop on Hampton Boulevard and 41street. Right in front of McDonalds. It was 9:00am the bus came 40 minutes later. I was upset about that. I call myself coming out early so I could be on time and the bus is running late. I get to Little Creek and Hampton Boulevard at 10:00am but the connecting bus wont come to 45 minutes after the hour so I decided to walk. There was a white boy who got off the bus too. He was trying to get to a new job that he was starting. I told him we can walk together. By the time we get down the other end he could catch the connecting bus on Grandy street. We walked straight down Little Creek together.

I got to my wife's block by 10:30am. I told him,

"You only got a five minute walk from here and you should be good." He said,

"Thanks for showing me where to go, have a nice day."

I walked up to the apartment. I could hear Shereef crying.

I went up the steps and knocked on the door.

Sonita answered.

"Who is it?"

I said, "It's me Sonita."

She opened the door. She had a knife in her hand and she looked upset.

I spoke, "Oh you're gonna stab me now. I'm sorry I'm a half an hour late. The bus was late so I walked here from Hampton Boulevard."

As she walked away I saw Shereef sitting in the car seat in the middle of the floor crying. Jehdiah was standing by the couch smiling; Abijah was sitting on the couch watching T.V. Sonita walked over to the other couch and sat down.

Jehdiah ran towards me and jumped in my arms. Abijah followed suit and Shereef was trying to get out of the car seat.

I hugged and kissed them. Then I put them down so I could get Shereef out of the car seat. As I was doing this I asked Sonita.

"Are you about to leave?"

She said, "No! I'm sick of him crying, so I locked him in the car seat."

When I took him out he was soak and wet. I told her.

"I see why he is crying he's soaked and wet. He's probably hungry too." She said to me,

"Well you attend to him; I'm off now that you're here."

I took him to the bedroom and changed him. Jehdiah and Abijah assisted me. Then we walked to the kitchen. I fixed him a bottle. Afterwards, we walked in the front room where Sonita was and sat on the couch across from her. I said to her,

"It's a beautiful day outside Sonita, lets take their bikes out and talk on the porch." She said sarcastically,

"I don't want to go out side! Let's talk about us."

I said," Well what about us?"

She said," See you don't care."

I said, "Sonita please I told you why I was late."

In the meantime I got up and I started pulling the boys bikes out this made them happy. They were jumping up and down then Sonita screamed on them,

"Stop all that noise; go in the room right now!"

Jehdiah and Abijah started crying and ran into the room.

I went back there and told them, "You don't have to. Come on with daddy." They came back out with me. But they stopped by the end of the couch. Right between the kitchen and the front room.

I walked back over to Sonita and I sat down. Shereef was finishing up his bottle so I put him in his walker. I told her,

"Look Sonita, I got my half of the rent for you."

She said, "I don't need it I got it covered."

I asked her, "Who did you get the money from?"

She answered, "Don't worry about it."

I said to her," No, I want to know."

She retorted," What do you care, you couldn't come here last night when I asked you." I said,

"Sonita I told you I had something to do.

I got the $50.00 dollars for the babysitter then."

She said, "I already paid her in advance so she is straight."

I said," Well I'm here now I can baby-sit the boys for you while you go to work tonight." She replied,

"Love I'm tired of that job, I'm quitting."

I asked her," Why? I told you I got you."

She blurted out," Love where was you at last night!? huh huh?"

I told her, "If you must know, I got me a room. That way if you wild out on me I got a place to stay." She screamed out,

"What! You got a room? So your free right! You can just do what you want! Just go on with life huh?" I calmly said,

"No, Sonita that's not true I'm here with ya'll I'm not going no where. But if you start bugging out I will have me a place to sleep in peace."

Then the phone rang and Sonita answered it. She said,

"Hey what's up?" The person must've said, "can you braid my hair?" because she said," I can't braid it today I got to go to work, but the way I feel I might don't go."

I had cut in and said, "Yes you are." Then she looked at me all mean and kept talking. Smiling she now said, "I'm off tomorrow maybe we can hook up then." I took Shereef out the walker and I sat next to her.

She was twirling the knife on her finger. I tried to reach for it and she pulled back.

The conversation went on for about another minute then she hung up.Out the blue she just started crying tears are falling down her face nonstop and she says "You know what, I don't even care anymore."

Jehdiah walked over to her side and said.

"It's gonna be okay mommy, daddy is here." Then he kissed her on her cheek and hugged her. Abijah came over and kissed her too. Then they both climbed up on the couch between us so I moved over closer to her. I started rubbing her shoulders. I had Shereef in my right arm and Jehdiah and Abijah were on my left leaning on Sonita, while her feet were stretched across the couch landing in my lap.

She whipped away her tears and started smiling. We all were smiling back at her. I said,

"See baby it's not all that bad." She said,

"Love, I'm tired I just can't take it no more, you know what. Just leave and take the boys with you. Go please go."

I asked her," Are you sure?"

With her voice cracking she said, "Go, all of you."

We bear hugged each other then I said,

"O.k. boys come on lets go outside and play, get your sneakers!"

The boys yelled, "Yeah! Where going with daddy!"

I got up and I started looking for Shereef things.

Then Sonita snapped and said, "You know what, never mind. YOU GO, LEAVE THE BOYS HERE!" I said,

"Come on Sonita you know they are gonna cry, we haven't been together for awhile." She said,

"You just don't care, get the fuck out or I'm a call the cops Now!"

I yelled back," I just got here!!"

She screamed even louder," Leave Love!"

Jehdiah started crying real hard. It was a scary cry. Waving his hand he said,

"I want to go with you daddy, come on." He reached for me to pick him up.

But Sonita intervened." Go in the room!"

Jehdiah wouldn't he stayed there crying putting his hands up for me to pick him up. Then Abijah started crying too.

Sonita took Shereef out my arms and put him in the walker.

Then she opened the door and told me to get out.

I walked out. I didn't want to argue with her or have her call the cops. She slammed the door behind me. I walked down the steps and I can here the children crying. As I got out the door I looked up to the window, Jehdiah and Abijah was in the window saying,

"Daddy come back, come back daddy!"

I told them, "Look your mother is bugging out sons. I'll see you tomorrow after school."

Jehdiah nodded his head, "No daddy come back!"

Sonita then appeared in the window and pulled them out and shut it. I started walking away. The boys then ran to the next window to see me pass by. I waved bye and Jehdiah nodded his head "No daddy don't leave me, come back!"

Sonita pulled them out of the window again. I turn my head and started walking back to the bus stop.

I ended up catching the bus back to Hampton Blvd. I had a 45 minute wait, so I went inside Popeye's to eat and study my barber book. I was in a daze the whole time. I couldn't believe she put me out and I just got there. The bus came and I went back to my room. My landlord was shocked to see me because I told him I was staying with my wife and children and I would probably be back later on in the week. He asked me, "What happen?"

I told him, "She is bugging out, so I left."

I rested for a while, and then I went to Sam's house and asked him did he have any other beats I could listen to. I wanted to write another song. He said, "Yeah, and Danielle is coming over."

I said, "Word, well we can work on something together. Ya'll can come over my place."

I stayed in his house while, he walked down the street to meet her.

Sam liked Danielle a lot. He wanted to show her how much of gentlemen he was. Once they got back, Sam got his music and we went to my place to work on new music all day and night. Afterwards Sam walked Danielle home and I went to sleep.

Monday September 30, 2002 I got up and ate breakfast. Then I watch TV. After that I went to Sam house. I called Sonita but no one answered the phone. I figured she went to the beach to see her cousins. I knew she had to be back at least by 3:00pm to pick Jehdiah up so my goal was to meet her at Jehdiah school.

I walk there from Sam house. I got there around 3:20.

Parents were leaving with their children; other children were waiting on their parents. Jehdiah wasn't there I figured she had picked him up already. I stayed out there until 4:00pm. I walked back to my room. I called again I got no answer. Samad came through and we got drunk. Finally he left to go home and I went to sleep.

Tuesday, October 1, 2002, I went to work and started cutting.

Around 2:00pm I get a call from the dude Sonita said was harassing her. "Yo Love what's up?"

I said," Who is this?"

He said, "It's Mike with the c.d.s and movies, Yo, you don't stay up here no more?" I said,

"Dig son its none of your business if I'm there or not. My wife told me how ya'll be pushing up on her. Listen leave my wife alone!"

He said, "Naw Love it ain't me it's them other dudes!"

I said, "I don't care who it is, leave her alone and I don't need anything from you. So don't come by my home you dig?"

He said,"Yo, I got you player."

Then I hung up. 4:00pm came by and Jehdiah didn't walk through the door. I'm thinking Sonita must be real mad at me. She haven't brought my sons to see me. Around 6:00pm I called the house the phone just rang. Damn she wont pick up. Fuck it she got to go to work tonight. I'll call her at her job. I got off at 8:00pm; got me a beer, and then I went to my room. Sam and Bryant came by. They chilled with me until about 12:00am that night. Afterwards, they left.

I called her job. Her coworker picked up the phone.

She said, "Hello This is Texaco how can I help you?"

I said, "Yes this is Randell, can I speak with Sonita please?"

Sarcastically she said, "Sonita? look she aint here.!!"

I calmly said," Listen stop playing with me I know she is there; can you put her on the phone?"

With a nasty attitude she continued, "I told you she aint here, and she didn't come in Sunday either.

I don't know what ya'll going through but ya'll need to get it together because she's about to get fired!"

Agitated, I said,"Ho, Ho, Ho, first of all what we are going through is none of your business, and she should be there!"

She said," Well she ain't and tell her if she don't come in tonight she won't have a job bye." click.

I know this bitch ain't just hang up on me. Something aint right I'm going over there right now. I know she didn't quit for real.

I asked the guy named Monte` to take me over to her place.

But he was too drunk to drive so I caught the cab.

The cab driver was real cool. He was talking about his women problems and he had me cracking up in the cab.

Then all of a sudden when he turned down my wife block, I saw police cars, fire trucks, and ambulances all over the place.

There was yellow tape going from the building out to the street.

My heart jumped and a lump formed in my neck. I jumped out of the cab while he was still driving. He blew the horn "Hey, you didn't pay me fell!!"

I ran back to give him $20 dollars and said, "keep the change."

I ran back towards the building and some Detectives stopped me from going in the building. They said,

"Hold up sir you can't go in there this is a crime scene."

I frantically said" What!! What are you talking about?"

He asked me," Who are you?"

I replied, "I'm Randell Barkley, and why are you preventing me from going in the building?"

He said," Listen calm down Mr. Barkley we need you to sit down." I said,

"I don't want to sit down, for what? What the fuck is going on?"

I look up to the window and I can see that someone is taking pictures in the apartment. The detectives start walking me back towards their car.

They calmly said,

"Listen Mr.Barkley we need you to come with us."

I asked, "Why?" My head is pounding, my legs are shaking, my heart is racing, and my blood pressure is rising.

He said," I don't know how to tell you but, **Your wife and three children are dead!**

A pain went through my soul so severe I couldn't breathe correctly. The words he said felt like I just got hit in the head with a steel bat. Everything went blank. I felt like I was in the Twilights Zone. They were talking to me but I couldn't hear them.

All I could think of was the last day that I was there, and seeing my children in the window begging me to stay.

He said,"Mr Barkley? Mr Barkley? are you alright?"

I screamed, "**Uh hell no! Hell no, I'm not alright!!!!!**

What the fuck happened? What do you mean they are dead? How?" He said,

"We don't know how? It's still under investigation."

"**You don't know how? Then how do you know they are dead? What happened, was it a fire? Were they shot? Or stabbed? Tell me something! This can't be happening! this is not true, you got the wrong people! My family ain't dead!!**

He said, "Calm down Mr. Barkley I'm sorry; the cause of death has not been established. By the way do you have any dental records on your wife?" I asked in shock,

"**Dental records? What the fuck are you talking about dental records for? What happened to my wife?** By now I'm hysterical, shaking inside and my heart is beating fast.

"**I know how my wife looks! What happened to her?**

He said, "Listen we need you to come down to the precinct with us. We need you to identify the bodies." I said,

"Oh no!!! I can't believe this shit!!! Hold up, it's a black book on the shelf could you get it for me please."

He said," Where is it?"

I said," On the shelf on the left hand side. Her family's phone numbers and address is in there. I got to notify her family. Something isn't right, its not right!"

"O.k. Mr Barkley could you have a seat please."

I sat down in the car. My head was pounding out of control. The first thing that came to my mind was calling her job to curse that Bitch out who hung up on me. I let her have it over the phone.

Then I called my brother Dawu up in New Jersey and told him what was going on. He told me to keep him on the phone so he could hear what the detectives was saying to me. My whole world was destroyed. This had to be a dream. This can't be true. not my wife. not my children.........

They took me to the precinct and ask me when was the last time I seen my wife and kids. I told them everything they wanted to know. I was crying so hard inside. I couldn't let these people see me in shambles so I was holding it in the best way I could.

After I answered all their questions I asked them again.

"You still didn't tell me what happened. I need to know!

I know my wife told me she was having problems with our neighbor friends harassing her lately. Come to think of it some dude called me at work asking me if I still lived with my wife.

Please tell me what happen!?!!"

He said,"Mr Barkley another detective will be in shortly to answer your questions. Just hang out in here. Can I get you something?"

"No, I don't want nothing but some answers."

About 20 minutes later the detective comes in and says "Mr. Barkley we got a call Monday morning stating that a lady was broke down on Campostella Bridge. Two different callers said she was alone. Her hazards were on. Once we arrived at the scene no one was there. We ran the plates and found out who the car belonged to, so we went back tracked to locate your wife.

Apparently she jumped off the bridge."

I screamed out," Jump off the bridge!!! Get the FUCK out of here with that bullshit. My wife ain't gonna jump off no bridge?!

For one, she can't swim. She aint gonna do no stupid shit like that! You expect me to believe that!

Another officer cut in and said," She wasn't trying to swim!"

Then the other detective intervened and said, "Woe, Woe watch what the fuck you're saying man, this is his wife idiot!"

I wanted to grab the officer pistol so bad and shoot the officer who made that comment. I knew I couldn't do anything about it.

I just stared at him with the look of death in my eyes.

The first detective continued to tell me how they found her body but her face was beyond recognition. That's why they wanted her dental records to identify her.

I told him, "She has a mark on her right leg from when she was small. But still that don't explain what happen to my children.

What's going on?"

"Mr. Barkley we believe your wife murdered them and then committed suicide."

With disbelief I yelled out, **Oh hell no! My wife loved our kids. Somebody else had to do this! You got it all wrong. My wife would never do such a thing!**

Our marriage wasn't that bad, we loved each other.

Matter of fact our new baby, was due on our anniversary!

Ya'll trying to tell me my wife did this, **Hell no! I don't believe it! It's no way!**"

He said," Listen Mr. Barkley again you have my condolences. I can only imagine how hard this is for you, but in a couple of hours we need you to identify their bodies. Now, I want you to understand something. They are not gonna look like they did when they were alive. They have been dead for a couple of days. You think you can handle it?"

In a sobbing tone I said," I don't know."

The next morning they took me to view my family. It was the longest ride ever. The sun was shining yet I couldn't see or hear a thing. All I could picture was my family and all the fun times we shared. The last 12 days was flashing before me.

certain things she said.

I walked through a door and the detective told me." We are gonna let you see the kids first. If you can't handle it we will let you look at a picture of your wife, and we will have her brought in covered up so you could identify the scar on her leg okay?"

"Okay." They pulled the curtains back and it was the most horrible sight I had ever seen. They look beaten up bad!

Jehdiah face was discolored with a few bruises. He was sucking on his lip. That's what he does when he goes to sleep. Abijah's head was swollen, his left eye was busted and his jaw was bruised up and swollen terrible.

Shereef looked like some one had choked him to death!!!

I screamed out, "What the fuck happened to them, they look like they were beaten up!! My legs were about to give out on me but I couldn't break in front of these people. I was trying not to cry but the tears escaped easily down my face. I was dead at that moment. My babies layed motionless on that table. All that ran through my head was Jehdiah begging me not to leave him. I wasn't there to fight for my babies. I left them to the mercy of their mother.

He said,"Mr. Barkley? Mr Barkley? are you alright?"

"Uh, Naw I'm fucked up right about now. I don't want to see anymore." Then he said,

"We still need you to identify your wife. I'm a hand you the picture."

When he handed me the picture and I looked at her, my heart felt like a thousand needles was puncture in it.

My wife had **No face, it was gone! No nose or lips, just eyes and teeth.** She looked **scared, like she seen a ghost.** My hands started shaking profusely.

I felt like throwing up and I couldn't take no more. Yet, they still needed me to identify the scar on her leg. Afterwards I went out of the morgue into the lobby and cried like a new born baby.

It hit me **Your entire family is gone! And it's nothing you can do about it! You should've stayed there, you should've stayed!**

The detectives drove me to my room. Then left. I cried my heart out to the point I had a terrible headache. I was in shock.

I was hoping I would wake up and it was all a dream. But it was FOR REAL. Now I'm in this room ALL BY MY SELF..........

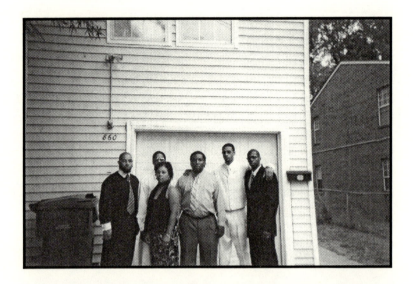

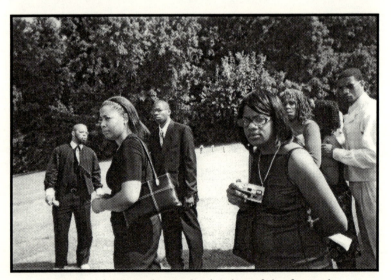

My brother's and sister's, the day of the funeral.

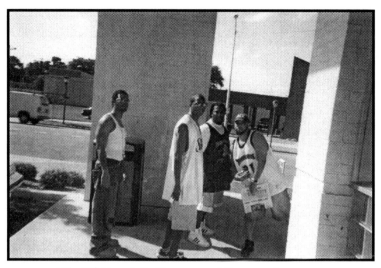

Khalif, Randell, Dawu, and Ibn, at the store.

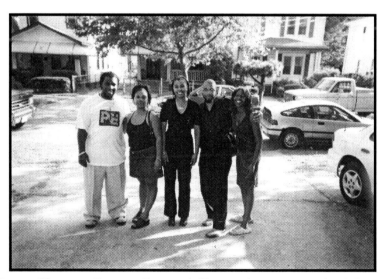

Dawu, Sherone, Fatima, Ibn, and Christie leaving to go back home.

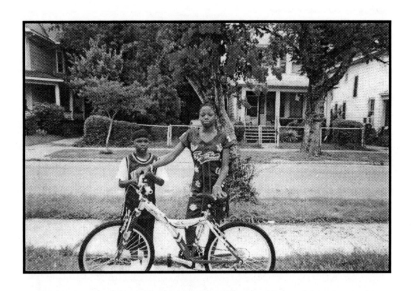

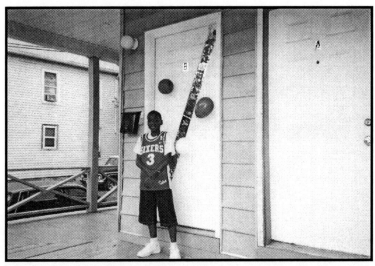

RAHSHON NAQUASHA, AND RANDELL JULY19,2003

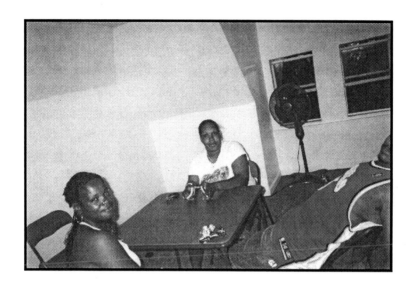

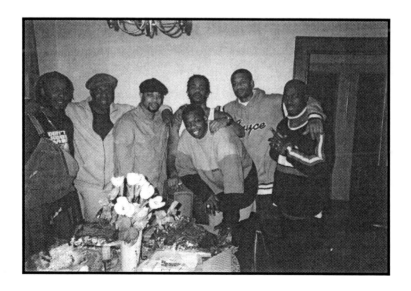

By that afternoon it was all over the news. No one could believe it. Not even me. Samad came through to console me. I was in pieces. I felt helpless. I thought to myself Sonita didn't even give it a chance. How could she give up on us? We been together for 8 and a half years. It's no way it could all end like this? Her love and conviction for this conclusion is beyond my understanding. Something had to be going on with her deeper than what I could've known. But what? I called my job and told my boss the deal. He suggested I get in contact with Wavy News 10 to help me at least raise money to bury my family. Society portrayed her as a struggling mother whose husband wasn't there for her and she went crazy. But my wife was a loving beautiful woman, and I was there to the last day.

So how could this happen?

I sat in the house pondering on these questions along with my brother Samad. Meanwhile the news came on and it shows them taking my sons out the apartment in white sheets. That turn my stomached and gave me an immediate headache. Chills ran through my body. Then the reporter said "the boys were drowned in their bathtub by their mother." I flipped out. "What! how do they know what happened and the detective's claim they didn't know?" I called the detective and asked him "Was it true? My sons were drowned?"

He said," Yes they were. At the time we had to get confirmation from the autopsy. I'm sorry you had to hear about it on the news, I was gonna call you. Look I'm a come by and get a statement from your landlord on when you moved in. I'm a need Sam and Danielle address as well."

"That's no problem." I gave him what he needed and then I hung up.

I contacted her uncle Robert and told him the little that I knew. I gave him my where about and told him to give the information to Annette, Kim, and Billy. After that I cried.

Samad told me our friends from Eternity had some money for me and told me to keep my head up. I have their full support.

I was in a whirlpool of pain. It didn't make any sense for Sonita to go to this extent. For what? What the hell was wrong with her? I just couldn't pin point it. Wavy News 10 came by for an interview with me. I really didn't know what to say. But one thing was for sure I wasn't going to break. I'm too much of an inside person. If I had to break it would be by myself or in the presence of my family. This situation here just crushed my will to live. I didn't want to be here no more. I was heart broken and the only way I saw me relieving the pain is by **My death. I never** felt this way before, **ever.**

Over the course of the next couple of days, my family piled in from everywhere. New Jersey, New York, Hawaii, Florida, Connecticut, Philadelphia, Atlanta, and North Dakota.

Just to see their faces was so encouraging for me. I realized then how much I was still **Loved** regardless of what my wife had done.

My family stayed away and supported me when I moved away from everybody just to be with Sonita and our children. They felt like if it made me happy they were fine with it. Now they are all here. Some I haven't seen in years. My landlord Mitch extended the rooming house to my family. It was a six family rooming house, three stories high. We occupied five of the rooms, that way my brothers, sisters, and cousins could be close to me.

They all knew how fragile I was at this time.

One of my clients told me to go through Metropolitan Funeral Home. It was right off Grandy Street. The President Kenneth Alexander was a very nice guy. He could see the pain and shock I was dealing with, as we went through setting the funeral up.

Sonita's Aunt Annette tried to take over and change everything we went through, although neither she nor the family were contributing any money towards the bill. That was frustrating. They were making all these demands and weren't offering a penny.

Once her cousin Billy found out, he came straight to me.

My family greeted him with love and hugs. Then he and I rolled out to talk. I told him what went down and we cried in each other's arms. He gave me some history on how Sonita's mother and grandparents services were held at their church, and closure for his family, would be held there.

Out of respect for him, plus the love and support he showed me the whole 8 and a half years I been with his cousin. I granted his wishes.

The morning of the Funeral I felt my sickest. I was throwing up, in a daze, and floating on fumes. I haven't eaten since I found out. My family got together and prayed. Once the limos came, we took pictures and left. It was a little conversation going on. When we arrive there it was packed with people. Wavy News 10 was there. When we got out the first person I saw was Billy. We hugged and my brothers came over to help carry the caskets alongside Sonita's Uncles. When they pulled out Shereef's casket I lost it. I immediately turned around and was heading for the limo. The tears and pain was enormance. My older female cousins and aunts surrounded me holding me.

I was shaking like an uncontrollable leaf. They told me,

"Calm down and get it together it's alright to cry."

We stood there for about ten minutes then I wiped my face and went towards the church door. Sonita's Aunt held my right hand and my cousin Keisha held my left. We walked in and both families followed suit. We sat down and the preacher preach, however I didn't hear a word he was saying. All I could do was stare at the caskets which held the **Love** of my **Life** and **Four** of my **Babies**. Once the session was over we left and went to the burial grounds. We formed a line and started walking to the burial site.

Ironically, the only seat that was available for me was right next to Janelle, Sonita's sister I met her through. I sat there, listen to the preacher preach and they were lowering my family in the ground. At that moment I knew, I was gonna **Kill Myself**.

I just sat there while everybody went back to their cars.

My brother Dawu sat next to me and said,

"Yo Hak, it's time to go."

Then I got up and started walking back to the limo.

I saw her aunt and she held my hand along with my brothers and sisters and I said a prayer with them. I felt heaven open its doors to my family at that second. Then we all went our separate ways. On the ride back to my room it was dead silence.

My family cooked and reminisced while I was in the room with my brother Kasseem and my sister Sherone. The pain was intensified a thousand times over. I couldn't talk about it without crying. Flashbacks of that last day weighed heavy on me. I was shocked, confused, disappointed, hurt, in turmoil, mad and I felt guilty for leaving...

My family stayed for a week, and then they left to go home. That's when my demons started attacking me night and day. I started getting high again to numb the pain. I was having nightmares. Plus I was hallucinating. I'd blank out and wake up across town. I started losing my mind. Praying for death...

November came around and I was in shock. The desire to die became realer and stronger everyday. I got in contact with Vernon and he paid for me to go to Hawaii. Just so I could get out of V.A. I had a great time. It was a reality check. This is a place we wanted to move to. One day Vernon and I went out to lunch with two beautiful sisters. We were at the mall. We ordered a seafood platter. While we were talking a picture caught my eye. I knew at that moment this was one of the places Sonita ate at. I could tell from the pictures she took. I immediately called Sonita on the phone. The phone kept ringing and ringing, and then I realized she was DEAD. My everything was GONE. Tears just pour down my face like Niagara Falls.

The women didn't know what was wrong with me. Vernon went ahead and explained to them. Afterwards, they took me back to his house. No matter how far away I was, the pain was still there.

Four days later I left and came back to V.A.

I stayed in Portsmouth with my sister. I was having nightmares every night. Waking up in cold sweats was a daily routine.

My brothers in New Jersey invited me up for thanksgiving.

I went and I got high as hell. All I wanted to do was get drunk. Anything that would numb the pain I was with it. We went out and partied but deep inside my heart moan. I stayed for a week, and then I left and came back to V.A.

In December I was a walking time bomb. Any little thing ticked me off and I wanted to fight.

By January I couldn't take it no more. I wanted out, so on January 3, 2003 I went and got a life insurance policy. I stuck it in my sister's room and put it in her name. I got me some drugs and beer and I set out to kill myself.

I went to a friend of mine and told him," I got beef with some one and I need your gun. I'll bring it back when I'm finish." Then he said,

"No Love, who are you beefing with? I'll go with you, but I'm not giving you a gun." I begged him but he wouldn't do it.

I left him and went riding around Norfolk trying to find some one else. I ended up in Champions Night club to holla at my friends from Eternity. They were happy to see me. However I knew this day was the last they would see me. They bought me beer and they introduce me to women. I dance a little, played some pool. Then I asked a couple of them for their gun. But No one would give it to me. They all were with the ride, but not with giving me their weapon. Around 1:30 am my sister calls me.

She is in New Jersey as well as my brother Samad. She said,

"Love, where are you at?" I told her,

"I 'm out in about why?" She continued,

"Jug said you told him about your life insurance policy and it's in my name. What's wrong with you?"

I couldn't hold it in no more. I had been fronting out in public for the last three months so I broke down in the bathroom.

"Look sis I love you, but I can't take it no more, I can't deal with this pain. I'm losing my fucking mind!! Give the family my love I'm out!!!" Franticly she said,

"No Randell don't hang up the phone, where are you? Don't do this!" I said,

"I'm sorry sis bye." click.

My heart started pumping real fast I could hear my children crying in my head saying," Daddy come with me! Daddy don't leave, come back, and come back!" I stormed out of the bathroom. Tears was falling down my face nonstop. I grabbed my coat and headed out the club.

People was looking at me but I kept walking. It was time for me to go. My head was pounding out of control. I was hearing Sonita's voice saying, "I don't care no more!"

And I was talking back, "Neither do I!"

My phone was ringing it was my cousin Rena. I picked up and all I could hear was," Randell where are you?

Where are you talk to me!!!"

I hung up the phone and got into my car. Tears was coming down so hard I could barely see in front of me. The phone rang again this time it was my brothers. "Hakeem don't do this where are you bro? What's going on, talk to us, we Love you don't leave us! I hung up and cried even harder. I sat in Champions Parke lot for ten minutes. I drank the rest of my beer and I put the car in drive. I screamed out, "Here I come Sonita I'm a see you tonight!"

I drove down Bramelton up to the Campostella Bridge Cutting through traffic. Once I got over the bridge I rode back up to the very spot my wife was at and park. I got out and said to my self "Fuck life."

I got on the bannister to go on the other side and at that moment I let go. Some one grabbed me and screamed!" Please don't jump!!!"

I turned around to see who was holding me. To my surprise, it was my cousin Keisha with tears in her eyes.

She said, "Don't do it cuz, not in front of my children!!!

Don't do it please." I screamed out,

"How did you find me?! What are you doing here! Let me die! Just let me go!"

She said in a crying tone, "My daughter woke up in the middle of the night and told me to drive to the bridge. She said you were at the bridge. So I jumped in my van and drove from the beach here."

I looked towards her van, and her children were in the window crying screaming no!!!! At that moment their faces turn into my children faces and I blanked out.

I was rushed to the hospital by the police. When I regain my consciousness I saw Billy Sonita's cousin. Then, my cousin. The nurse who came to check my presser look like my dead grandmother and I blanked out again. I woke up hours later. I was in a room where I was confined for four days. On the 8th floor with the crazy people. All I did was cry and sleep all day. I just couldn't accept the fact my wife done this to me. Why? For what? How could she feel this way and do such a terrible thing. Sonita knew I loved her and our children unconditionally. What's the reason? What was she going through?

Once I was release from the hospital I had to follow up with a shrink. They gave me a prescription that kept me up at night. I had the shakes. Plus I was still hurt. The desire to kill myself hung heavy over my head. Life seemed so pointless without my family. The shrinks couldn't help me. He said," Your situation is very complicated. Try to find you some one else."

I really was lost, because no one could seem to relate. Then the medicine was to expensive. I was force to stop using it. I went back to the only thing I knew, a forty and a blunt.

One day out of the blue I get a call at my sister house, it was Susan. She found out four months later what happened. We talked on the phone for the first time in five years. She shared with me everything that was going on with our children and she said, "They want to see you." I was happy about that. I went to Brooklyn to see her and my children. It was one of the happiest days of my life. She let them live with me to help me recover from the lost of my other children. However I still was incomplete inside. I needed help. I went to see another shrink. The shrink was a cool old guy. His office was out in Virginia Beach. He was very compassionate and frank with me when he said, "You have the right to feel however you feel. If you are mad, happy, or sad. I'm not the one to tell you, that's wrong. The average person doesn't experience such a dramatic loss like you. Here is your money back. You might want to seek out another psychiatrist. I don't know what to tell you."

I felt lost and confused again. The only thing I could think of was to research Post Partum Depression for my self. I needed answers and what I found out blew my mind. In one book titled "Stop Depression Now" on page 190 it states." Postpartum Depression leads some women to feel inadequate as mothers, fearful for their children, and unable to maintain their other relationships. In severe cases it can lead to obsessive compulsive disorder, in which a mother <u>cannot let go of thoughts of harm coming to her child, sometimes even from herself.</u> Thoughts which shock and depress her still more."

In the later part of the paragraph it states," If you were depress following one birth your more likely to <u>suffer again with subsequent births.</u> The major contributor is <u>stress.</u>

I never knew this and I've been married twice, with a total of ten children. It was like a veil was removed from my eyes.

This explains the mood swings.

Then, in another book called "Women and Depression" Chapter 11 page 133 states, "You are at an increased risk of experiencing postpartum depression if you:

1. Have a <u>history</u> of Depression.
2. Experience depression during <u>pregnancy</u>
3. Experience <u>marital problems.</u>
4. Undergo <u>difficult</u> life events during <u>pregnancy</u>
5. <u>Lack</u> a social system."

All five categories was my wife. I was all my wife had. Her world was over once she put me out. That's why she begged me to come back. She really didn't know what she was going through, and without me she wasn't trying to go through it alone.

I wish this information was readily available for us. This whole Tragedy could've been avoided...

I was a second away from death, but Jehovah God spared me so I can share light and help millions to maintain Life.

It's nothing in this world I wouldn't give just to have her back in my life. She was a great and wonderful woman who was victimized by an illness she knew nothing about. But I will not let her voice go unheard. Sonita represents all woman who go through this common thing called birth, yet she wasn't educated on the common thing called POST PARTUM DEPRESSION or POST PARTUM PSYCOSIS.

In our society we need to be aware of this just like CANCER and AIDS. So as long as I live I will pursue this issue and bring it to the light.

Here are some symptoms and remedies for yourself or someone you love, if they are suffering from depression.

Along with hypertension, high cholesterol and diabetes, depression is considered a risk factor for heart disease.

Physiologically depression affects the amount of stress hormones in the body which makes the blood vessels more ragged and prone to forming plaque'.

A remedy for this problem is to seek counseling. (something my wife wasn't aware of)

The longer depression goes untreated, the more damage is done to your blood vessels which makes seeking help sooner rather than later of paramount importance. Help is available through communication, counseling, therapy, and medication. You may be an independent person like my wife, and deal with your issues alone, but this is one time you should seek HELP.

Other factors may cause depression that may need treatment.

Chronic stressor whether it's about the boss, the bills, your mate, or racial bias. Unrelenting anxiety puts the body in a "constant state of emergency" High levels of stress hormones such as cortisol and adrenaline, which are needed for your fight or flight response get pumped into your system. Being though there no actual danger for which a fight or flight is needed, the chemicals are left to circulate through your system doing damage.

They raise blood pressure and make blood platelets more sticky and damaging to the lining of the blood vessels.

This in turn can initiate inflammation thus increasing the risk of forming clots.

If you are dealing with this, the best way to counter act this is by looking for effective outlets to release negative emotions and tension in your body. Chronic stress puts elevated amounts of these chemicals in the body, you need to burn them off. Aerobic exercise at least four times a week in 30 minute session will help. Walking, jogging, cycling, and swimming is good too.

Being angry and hostile are link to coronary artery disease.

One reason is frequent bouts of anger, increase heart rate, and raise blood pressure can form blood clots in the coronary arteries.

The best defense for this is a good offense. Walk away, get from the situation. That means becoming more aware of when you first begin to feel anger build up. (I left, but my wife was still upset)

Women have a tendency to <u>focus</u> on a problem and <u>ruminate</u> over it. That only prolongs the stress response rather than ease it.

If your inclination is to call your girlfriends and your mama and keep going over the problem, do it <u>once</u>, get it off your chest. Then let it go and occupy yourself in something else, positive and refreshing.

Avoid Isolating yourself. Forming a network of friends and love ones who care about you plus support you serves as a powerful buffer against the kinds of stress that can lead to making poor health choices and may contribute to developing disease.

Researcher believe that people who form solid social relationship tend to live longer, smoke less, eat a healthier diet and are more likely to have routine check ups. The best thing you can do also is go to the library, meditate, and pray to God, play cards, exercise. Reach out. Don't be afraid or embarrass to admit you need help. These are things I had to undergo myself, just to find myself. So I'm doing things that can help people in ways my wife wasn't able to get.

In loving memory of my wife. SONITA BARKLEY.
I LOVE YOU BABY, and I'LL SEE YOU IN THE NEXT LIFE.

Now 4 years later I have the BARKLEY GROUP which was formed in the memory of my family.

Its a non profit organization design to help people in seven areas.

1. Raise awareness about post partum depression and the detrimental effect it has on men and women as a whole.
2. Make sure this information is provided in all hospitals and clinics.
3. Set up a program where mothers can have a support system and provide food and shelter if needed.
4. The program will offer up home visitation for a year to women who has been diagnose with Post partum Depression or post partum psychosis.
5. A Hotline will be set up for woman who has homicidal or suicidal thoughts.
   At that time we would provide them with our services.
6. Shelter for the depress woman with children. Plus education for fathers to help assist their baby mothers.
7. Help people reach out to God for help, and strength to endure.

*WOMAN DON'T BE AFRAID TO PRAY
OR SHARE YOUR INNER FEELINGS
WITH YOUR MAN, DOCTORS OR NEXT
OF KIN. IT WILL BE WORTH IT, IF YOU
CAN GET HELP IN THE END.............*

*TAKE IT FROM ME,
A HEART BROKEN SOUL MATE.............*

THE END.

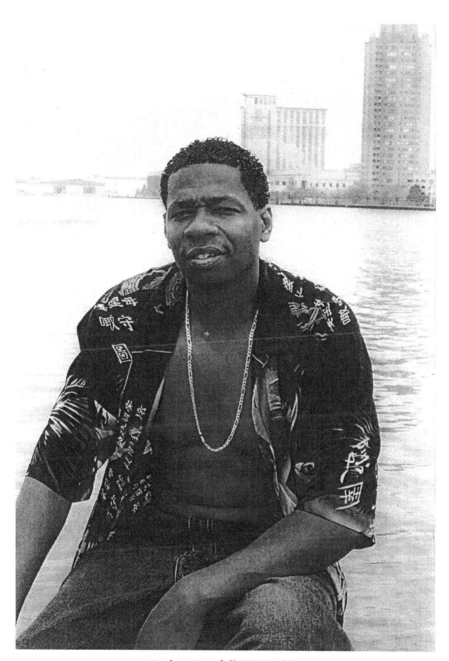
Author Randell W. Barkley